Assessing Essential Skills of Veterinary Technology Students

Assessing Essential Skills of Veterinary Technology Students

Third Edition

Edited by

Laurie J. Buell
Mercy College, Dobbs Ferry, NY, USA

Lisa E. Schenkel
Mercy College, Dobbs Ferry, NY, USA

and

Sabrina Timperman
Mercy College, Dobbs Ferry, NY, USA

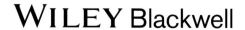

This edition first published 2017. © 2017 by John Wiley & Sons, Inc.

Editorial Offices
1606 Golden Aspen Drive, Suites 103 and 104, Ames, Iowa 50010, USA
The Atrium, Southern Gate, Chichester, West Sussex, PO19 8SQ, UK
9600 Garsington Road, Oxford, OX4 2DQ, UK

For details of our global editorial offices, for customer services and for information about how to apply for permission to reuse the copyright material in this book please see our website at www.wiley.com/wiley-blackwell.

Library of Congress Cataloging-in-Publication data applied for

ISBNs:
978-1-119-04211-2 [Paperback]
978-1-119-04212-9 [ePDF]
978-1-119-04213-6 [epub]

A catalogue record for this book is available from the British Library.

Wiley also publishes its books in a variety of electronic formats. Some content that appears in print may not be available in electronic books.

Cover image: (Left) Monty Rakusen/Gettyimages; (Right top) DenGuy/Gettyimages; (Right bottom) zoranm/Gettyimages
Cover design: Wiley

Set in 10/12pt Warnock by SPi Global, Pondicherry, India

Printed in Singapore by C.O.S. Printers Pte Ltd

10 9 8 7 6 5 4 3 2 1

Contents

Contributors *vii*
Preface *ix*
About the Companion Website *xi*

1   **Veterinary Management** *1*
     Sandra Bertholf
1.1   Procedures and Policies *1*
     Veterinary Management Skills Number 1–14
1.2   Communication Skills *3*
     Veterinary Management Skills Number 15–21
1.3   Ethics and Jurisprudence *3*
     Veterinary Management Skills Number 22–25
     References *4*

2   **Pharmacology** *5*
     Laurie J. Buell and Lisa E. Schenkel
2.1   Pharmacologic Fundamentals of Drug Administration *5*
     Pharmacology Skills Number 1–11
2.2   Pharmacy Essentials of Drug Dispensing *7*
     Pharmacology Skills Number 12–15
     References *8*

3   **Medical Nursing** *9*
     Deirdre Douglas, Laurie J. Buell and Lisa E. Schenkel
3.1   Assessment of the Veterinary Patient *9*
     Medical Nursing Skills Number 1–27
3.2   Nursing Care of the Veterinary Patient *12*
     Medical Nursing Skills Number 28–69
3.2.1   Husbandry of Common Domestic Species *12*
     Deirdre Douglas, Lisa E. Schenkel, Laurie J. Buell and Sabrina Timperman
     Medical Nursing Skills Number 28–36
3.2.2   Nutrition of Common Domestic Species *14*
     Deirdre Douglas, Lisa E. Schenkel, Sabrina Timperman and Laurie J. Buell
     Medical Nursing Skills Number 37–42
3.2.3   Therapeutics for Common Domestic Species *15*
     Lisa E. Schenkel, Laurie J. Buell, Sabrina Timperman, Nicole VanSant and Deirdre Douglas
     Medical Nursing Skills Number 43–69
3.3   Dental Procedures in Small Animals *21*
     Howard Gittelman
     Medical Nursing Skills Number 70–72
     References *23*

4   Anesthesia *25*
Laurie J. Buell and Lisa E. Schenkel

4.1   Perioperative Management of the Veterinary Patient *25*
        Anesthesia and Analgesia Skills Number 1–9

4.2   Management and Use of Anesthetic Equipment *30*
        Anesthesia and Analgesia Skills Number 10–22
        References *34*

5   Surgical Nursing and Assisting *37*
Laurie J. Buell and Lisa E. Schenkel

5.1   Fundamentals of Common Surgical Procedures *37*
        Surgical Nursing Skills Number 1–10

5.2   Experience with Common Surgical Procedures *39*
        Surgical Nursing Skills Number 11–12

5.3   Management of the Veterinary Surgical Patient *39*
        Surgical Nursing Skills Number 13–34

5.4   Management of Surgical Equipment and Facilities *44*
        Surgical Nursing Skills Number 35–44
        References *47*

6   Clinical Laboratory Procedures *49*
*Lisa E. Schenkel, Sabrina Timperman, Laurie J. Buell, Judy Duffelmeyer-Kramer,
Robin E. Sturtz and Deirdre Douglas*

6.1   Management of Laboratory Specimens and Equipment *49*
        Clinical Laboratory Procedures Skills Number 1–4

6.2   Diagnostic Laboratory Procedures *49*
        Clinical Laboratory Procedures Skills Number 5–48
        References *57*

7   Radiography *59*
Sandra Bertholf and Sabrina Timperman
        Radiography Skills Number 1–12
        Reference *62*

8   Laboratory Animal Care and Procedures *63*
Natalie H. Ragland
        Laboratory Animal Care and Procedures Skills Number 1–17
        References *67*

9   Avian and Exotic Animal Nursing *69*
Sabrina Timperman, Lisa E. Schenkel, Laurie J. Buell and Carol J. Gamez
        Exotic Animal Nursing Skills Number 1–10
        References *73*

Index *75*

Contributors

Sandra Bertholf, BS, LVT
Instructor
Veterinary Technology Program
Mercy College
Veterinary Technologist
Animal Medical of New City
New City, NY

Laurie J. Buell, MS, LVT
Veterinary Technologist
Former Associate Professor and Program Director
Veterinary Technology Program
Mercy College
Dobbs Ferry, NY

Deirdre Douglas, BS, LVT, VTS (ECC)
Veterinary Technologist
Former Adjunct
Veterinary Technology Program
Mercy College
Dobbs Ferry, NY

Judy Duffelmeyer-Kramer, AAS, LVT
Former Supervising Animal Health Technician
The Wildlife Conservation Society
Bronx, NY

Former Adjunct
Veterinary Technology Program
Mercy College
Dobbs Ferry, NY

Carol J. Gamez, DVM
Practice Owner, Veterinarian
Georgetown Veterinary Hospital
Georgetown, CT

Howard Gittelman, DVM, MS
Hospital Director
Animal Medical of New City
New City, NY

Natalie H. Ragland, DVM, cert LAM
Former Adjunct
Veterinary Technology Program
Mercy College
Dobbs Ferry, NY

Lisa E. Schenkel, DVM, CCRT, CVMA
Assistant Professor
Program Director
Veterinary Technology Program
Mercy College
Dobbs Ferry, NY

Associate Veterinarian
Animal Medical of New City
New City, NY

Robin E. Sturtz, DVM
Associate Veterinarian
The Cat Hospital
Williston Park, NY

Sabrina Timperman, DVM
Associate Professor
Associate Program Director
Veterinary Technology Program
Mercy College
Dobbs Ferry, NY

Nicole VanSant, BS, LVT, VTS (ECC)
Nursing Supervisor
Cornell University Veterinary Specialists
Stamford, CT

Adjunct
Veterinary Technology Program
Mercy College
Dobbs Ferry, NY

Preface

Veterinary technicians and technologists are highly educated and skilled professionals who team with veterinarians to offer state-of-the-art veterinary care. Clearly, to succeed in the increasingly complex and sophisticated fields of veterinary science and medicine, the veterinary technology student must learn solid technical skills. However, today's veterinary technology student also must develop the ability to make competent decisions based on knowledge of veterinary science and medicine as learned in the classroom and through practical experience. It is the role of the veterinary technology educator to help each student attain requisite skills, knowledge, and decision-making capabilities and, then, to evaluate each student's competencies.

At the same time, a wide variety of veterinary technology programs are educating future veterinary technicians and veterinary technologists. At this writing, there are 235 veterinary technology programs. Most are 2-year programs, but 24 are 4-year programs. Nine are on-line programs in which the veterinary technician educator may be thousands of miles away from the student (Committee on Veterinary Technician Education and Activities, 2016).

These facts present significant challenges in assessing the veterinary technology student. To some degree, the evaluation of any student's competency is inherently subjective, even when the performance of a technical skill is being assessed. How, then, does the veterinary technology educator take steps to minimize subjectivity when evaluating each student's ability to make informed judgments based on a strong foundation of knowledge? How does one define standards of competence in keeping with an entry-level veterinary technician? When comparing veterinary technology programs, how does one attempt to evaluate whether or not standards are at all consistent

or equivalent? One answer to these questions may lie in construction of explicit assessment criteria.

The Committee on Veterinary Technician Education and Activities (CVTEA©) of the American Veterinary Medical Association (AVMA) has issued a list of essential skills that must be satisfactorily accomplished and decision-making abilities that must be adequately developed by veterinary technology students. The goal of this third edition is to provide explicit, up-to-date assessment criteria for not only hands-on skills but also decision-making capabilities considered essential as of January, 2016 (Committee on Veterinary Technician Education and Activities, 2016).

The contributors to this text developed these criteria based on their experiences teaching in 4-year, Bachelor-of-Science degree, and 2-year, Associate-in-Applied-Science degree Veterinary Technology Programs, as well as in years of clinical practice. We are grateful to the contributors, who enthusiastically devoted their time and effort to the completion of this work.

It is our hope that this text will be of use, at least, in the following ways:

- To help provide students with clear guidelines as to what they are expected to learn and how they will be evaluated.
- To help provide educators with a more standardized means of assessing students' performance of skills, knowledge and abilities.
- To help provide students and educators in different veterinary technology programs with a means of comparing standards of competency.

Laurie J. Buell
Lisa E. Schenkel
Sabrina Timperman
June 2016

References

Committee on Veterinary Technician Education and Activities. (2016, January). *CVTEA Accreditation Policies and Procedures - Appendix I*. Retrieved from American Veterinary Medical Association: https://www.avma.org/ProfessionalDevelopment/Education/Accreditation/Programs/Pages/cvtea-pp-appendix-i.aspx (accessed September 14, 2016).

Committee on Veterinary Technician Education and Activities. (2016). *Programs accredited by the AVMA Committee on Veterinary Technician Education and Activities (CVTEA)*. Retrieved from American Veterinary Medical Association: https://www.avma.org/ProfessionalDevelopment/Education/Accreditation/Programs/Pages/vettech-programs.aspx (accessed September 14, 2016).

About the Companion Website

This book is accompanied by a companion website:

www.wiley.com/go/buell/skills

Instructions

This text is accompanied by an online list of skills, knowledge, and decision-making abilities considered essential for veterinary technologists and technicians by the CVTEA of the AVMA. (Committee on Veterinary Technician Education and Activities, 2016) For the purposes of this text, these items are collectively referred to as "skills" and are numerically organized within each chapter. The online list can be found at (http://to be entered once the url is established).

The intent of this text is to provide standard criteria for the assessment of each skill by veterinary technology program personnel.

In the online component, bold face test denotes hands-on (psychomotor) skills. These are also marked with a hand symbol (). Veterinary technology students are expected to physically perform these skills.

In addition, in the online component, the word "Group" follows certain skills. This indicates that the skill may be performed by a group of program students, but each student must actively participate in performing some aspect of the skill. Observation alone is not acceptable.

Students

In the online list of skills, please enter the course number(s) in which you satisfactorily accomplished, performed or developed the skill or ability, as well as the date of its assessment by your instructor. Also, print your instructor's name in the appropriate space. Once you have entered this information, your instructor must indicate your assessment for that skill and sign their name.

Veterinary Technology Program Personnel (Instructors)

Once the student has satisfactorily accomplished a skill, please enter your assessment in the appropriate space. To help guide your evaluation, this text defines the term "satisfactory" as meaning at a level consistent with a graduating veterinary technology student, who is entering the profession.

The accompanying text provides standard criteria to be used as guidelines in your assessment of the student. Each skill is numerically organized within each chapter. The number of each skill in the online list corresponds to the same number in the text.

In addition, once the student has satisfactorily accomplished a skill, please be certain to sign your full name in the appropriate space on the online skills list to indicate that the student has successfully accomplished the skill.

Reference

Committee on Veterinary Technician Education and Activities. (2016, January). *CVTEA Accreditation Policies and Procedures – Appendix I*. Retrieved from American Veterinary Medical Association: https://www.avma.org/ProfessionalDevelopment/Education/Accreditation/Programs/Pages/cvtea-pp-appendix-i.aspx (accessed September 14, 2016).

1

Veterinary Management

Sandra Bertholf

1.1 Procedures and Policies

1) **The student demonstrates the ability to participate in the day-to-day functioning of veterinary facilities in a manner that is helpful to clients, patients and the facility.**
   - The student demonstrates the ability to display professional demeanor and appropriate conduct at all times with clients, patients, and co-workers.
2) **The student shows understanding of how to efficiently schedule appointments as well as to effectively admit, discharge and triage patients by phone and in person.**
   - The student displays understanding of the importance of pleasant, professional, and appropriate communication with clients.
   - The student demonstrates appreciation of the importance of being responsive to the needs of the client, while following the guidelines and policies of the facility.
   - The student shows knowledge of how to schedule appointments and procedures correctly and precisely, following the guidelines and policies of the facility.
   - The student shows awareness of the importance of obtaining all necessary and appropriate patient information, including but not limited to, contact numbers, client concerns/requests, change in patient status, and so on. The student recognizes the significance of obtaining signed consent forms/treatment plans when appropriate.
   - The student shows understanding of the importance of clearly and accurately communicating proper at-home patient care and any other necessary follow-up care to clients.
   - The student displays knowledge of how to identify veterinary medical emergencies in a timely manner. The student recognizes the importance of responding appropriately and quickly triaging patients, as well as accurately obtaining and communicating vital information to the veterinarian.

3) **The student demonstrates understanding of how to correctly develop and maintain individual client/patient records, prepare vaccination certificates and other appropriate forms.**
   - The student shows knowledge of how to document the client's name, address, phone number, and email address, as well as thorough patient identification information, including species, breed, age, gender, reproductive status, coloring, markings, microchips, identification numbers, insurance information, and so on, in the medical record.
   - The student displays knowledge of appropriate veterinary medical terminology and abbreviations.
   - The student shows the ability to write legibly and use correct spelling and grammar.
   - The student demonstrates the ability to record information accurately, using correct formatting and following the guidelines and protocols of the facility.
   - The student displays appreciation of the veterinary medical record as a legal document. The student demonstrates awareness of the proper method of correcting an error by making a single line through the incorrect entry so that it is still legible, initialing and dating the change.
   - The student displays knowledge that altering a record in any other manner could be perceived as deceptive. The student demonstrates awareness that, alternatively, an addendum could be added to the record referring to the prior entry.
4) **The student demonstrates basic computer skills.**
   - The student correctly uses electronic communications and word-processing programs, displays information literacy, and so on.

Assessing Essential Skills of Veterinary Technology Students, Third Edition. Edited by Laurie J. Buell, Lisa E. Schenkel and Sabrina Timperman.
© 2017 John Wiley & Sons, Inc. Published 2017 by John Wiley & Sons, Inc.
Companion website: www.wiley.com/go/buell/skills

5) **The student demonstrates computer skills necessary for effective use of veterinary practice management and/or other computer software programs.**

- The student demonstrates understanding of patient veterinary medical record systems, including how to correctly enter new clients into patient record systems and how to properly develop patient records such as vaccination certificates, health certificates, and travel documents.

6) **The student displays knowledge of on-line veterinary services.**

- The student shows understanding of how to process on-line sample submission forms, submit on-line pharmacy requests, utilize veterinary learning communities, and complete on-line finance plan applications, and so on.

7) **The student demonstrates knowledge of how to properly file and retrieve medical documents and radiographs.**

- The student shows awareness of filing systems used at various facilities and how to correctly file and retrieve information, including but not limited to patient records, radiographs, clinical laboratory findings, surgical reports, and so on.

8) **The student demonstrates the ability to correctly prepare and maintain logs and records in accordance with regulatory requirements.**

- The student displays knowledge of record-keeping procedures in use at various facilities. The student shows the ability to complete and maintain all required logs and documentation in a manner that observes regulatory guidelines, including controlled substances, radiography, surgery, anesthesia, and laboratory logs.

9) **The student demonstrates understanding of how to effectively control inventory.**

- The student shows familiarity with computerized and/or manual systems that are aimed at ensuring that adequate supplies are available and stock is rotated, while expenses and/or losses are minimized.

10) **The student displays knowledge of pertinent governmental agencies and their regulations, as they apply to veterinary facilities and the practice of veterinary medicine and/or veterinary technology.**

- The student demonstrates understanding of the importance of compliance with the regulatory roles of OSHA, FDA, DEA, USDA, and so on, as they apply to the practice of veterinary medicine and/or veterinary technology.

11) **The student demonstrates awareness of proper procedures for disposal of hazardous materials.**

- The student displays knowledge of types of hazardous materials (including, but not limited to, developer solution, pesticides, chemotherapeutic agents, anesthetic gases, etc.), and biohazards (blood, cultures, isolation wastes, laboratory wastes, patient tissues, etc.).
- The student displays knowledge of the appropriate safety precautions for handling and storing hazardous materials and biohazards, including the use of personal protective equipment, in compliance with governmental regulations.
- The student demonstrates knowledge of proper disposal procedures for hazardous materials and biohazards (red bag waste), in compliance with governmental regulations.
- The student shows awareness of how to properly identify, handle, and dispose of sharps.

12) **The student demonstrates understanding of how to institute and follow appropriate sanitation and infection control procedures.**

- The student displays knowledge of potential routes of disease transmission.
- The student shows appreciation of the importance of developing, implementing, and adhering to appropriate sanitation/infection control protocols in all areas of the facility, including laboratory, patient, and staff areas.
- The student demonstrates knowledge of the appropriate use of personal protective equipment (PPE) in preventing disease transmission.
- The student displays knowledge of how to correctly identify patients that should be housed in isolation units.
- The student demonstrates knowledge of the proper use of isolation units. The student shows knowledge of how to implement and adhere to sanitation/infection control protocols including, but not limited to: cleaning, disinfection, sterilization, use of disinfectant foot baths, and the correct use of PPE.

13) **The student demonstrates knowledge of how to efficiently handle day-to-day financial transactions.**

- The student displays cognizance of representative bookkeeping procedures in place at veterinary facilities
- The student displays knowledge of how to utilize manual and electronic systems to process daily client-based financial transactions.
- The student displays the ability to explain the costs of quality veterinary care in a manner that reinforces the veterinarian's recommendations.

14) **Student shows knowledge of how to participate in the operations of veterinary facilities in a manner that is beneficial to clients, patients, and the facility.**
    - The student displays the ability to behave in a professional manner at all times.
    - The student shows appreciation for the importance of playing a valuable role as a member of the veterinary team.

1.2 Communication Skills

15) **The student demonstrates the ability to effectively communicate in written, oral, and electronic formats.**
    - The student displays awareness of how to use each communication mode appropriately, effectively obtaining and conveying information in a professional manner.

16) **The student demonstrates understanding of appropriate interpersonal skills and team dynamics.**
    - The student demonstrates the ability to interact with other team members in a cooperative, helpful and professional manner.
    - The student follows directions and responds positively to constructive criticism and uses it to improve performance.

17) **The student displays the ability to apply appropriate interpersonal skills in communicating with the public.**
    - The student shows understanding of the veterinary technician's/technologist's role in promoting the profession.
    - The student shows appreciation of the role of the veterinary technician/technologist in conveying the importance of quality care to the public.
    - The student demonstrates the ability to utilize professional etiquette in all communications with the public, including email and in person.

18) **The student demonstrates proper professional etiquette for telephone communications.**
    - The student demonstrates knowledge of how to clearly communicate with clients in a pleasant, professional and appropriate manner.
    - The student demonstrates appreciation of the importance of caring and being responsive to the needs of the client, while following the guidelines and policies of veterinary facilities.

19) **The student displays knowledge of the legal requirements for establishing and maintaining a valid veterinarian-client-patient relationship.**
    - The student shows knowledge of the criteria for a valid veterinary-client-patient relationship (Food and Drug Administration, 2014).

    - The student shows knowledge of the necessity for establishing a valid veterinarian-client-patient relationship prior to vaccination, as well as drug administration, dispensing and prescription.

20) **The student demonstrates the ability to educate clients at a level that is understandable to the client.**
    - The student shows the ability to communicate with clients appropriately and professionally, providing accurate information.
    - The student prepares clear, accurate educational handouts for clients, such as post-operative or bandage care instructions, discharge information, and so on.

21) **The student shows the ability to appropriately utilize crisis intervention and/or grief management skills when interacting with clients.**
    - The student demonstrates appreciation of the impact that serious illness and/or the death of a pet can have on a client.
    - The student displays familiarity with the various stages of the grieving process and shows the ability to appropriately discuss serious illness and/or death with client.
    - The student demonstrates knowledge of how to discuss the decision to euthanize in an appropriate manner with clients, showing due empathy and concern, while remaining professional.
    - The student demonstrates awareness of appropriate behavior with clients during and after euthanasia.
    - The student displays knowledge of how to recognize severe or abnormal grieving and shows familiarity with appropriate resources for professional assistance.

1.3 Ethics and Jurisprudence

22) **The student demonstrates clear understanding of and recognizes the necessity to observe laws pertaining to veterinarians and veterinary technicians/technologists.**
    - The student demonstrates knowledge and practical understanding of the applicable state practice act for veterinary technicians/technologists, in states where one exists.
    - The student displays knowledge of the applicable state practice act for veterinarians.
    - The student demonstrates knowledge and practical understanding of the code of ethics for veterinary technicians/technologists, as developed by the ethics committee of the National Association of Veterinary Technicians in America (NAVTA). (National Association of Veterinary Technicians in America, 2014)

23) **In all interactions with clients and staff members, the student demonstrates knowledge of how to behave professionally and ethically in light of legal boundaries.**
   - The student demonstrates appreciation of the potential legal ramifications of client and staff interactions.

24) **The student exhibits dedication to providing high quality patient care.**
   - The student demonstrates the requisite knowledge as well as motivation needed to provide high caliber patient care.
   - The student demonstrates appreciation of the importance of continuing education in providing high quality care.

   - The student displays recognition of the ethical responsibility to provide high quality patient care.

25) **The student displays understanding of how to maintain confidentiality as it pertains to client and patient information.**
   - The student demonstrates a clear understanding of the meaning of confidentiality as it pertains to clients and patients, recognizing its essential nature and respecting it at all times.
   - The student shows understanding of legal and ethical considerations regarding confidentiality.
   - As stated in the NAVTA Code of Ethics, the student protects "confidential information provided by clients" (National Association of Veterinary Technicians in America, 2014).

References

Food and Drug Administration. (2014, December 9). *Animal Medicinal Drug Use Clarification Act of 1994.* Retrieved May 10, 2016, from U.S. Food and Drug Administration: www.fda.gov/AnimalVeterinary/ GuidanceComplianceEnforcement/ ActsRulesRegulations/ucm085377.htm (accessed September 14, 2016).

National Association of Veterinary Technicians in America. (2014, December 11). *About NAVTA-National Association of Veterinary Technicians in America.* Retrieved May 10, 2016, from NAVTA.net: http://c.ymcdn.com/sites/www. navta.net/resource/collection/946E408F-F98E-4890-9894- D68ABF7FAAD6/navta_vt_code_of_ethics_07.pdf (accessed September 14, 2016).

2

Pharmacology

Laurie J. Buell and Lisa E. Schenkel

2.1 Pharmacologic Fundamentals of Drug Administration

1) **The student displays knowledge of how to correctly comply with the veterinarian's pharmacy (medication) orders, both written and verbal.**
   - The student displays understanding of the meaning of the terms "dose, dosage strength, dosage interval, and dosage (or dosage regimen)" and how to implement them correctly in the clinical setting.
   - The student shows knowledge of terms used in medication orders, including appropriate abbreviations, and how to apply them correctly in the clinical setting.
   - The student recognizes the importance of verifying patient identification, selecting the correct drug in the proper dosage form, and administering the prescribed dose via the appropriate route at the correct time.

2) **The student demonstrates knowledge of various drug categories, mechanisms of action, major therapeutic uses, and common, clinically significant adverse effects.**
   - The student demonstrates basic understanding of the clinical pathology underlying disease processes targeted by frequently used drugs.
   - The student demonstrates fundamental understanding of primary mechanisms of action of commonly used drugs. Based on this knowledge, the student displays the basic ability to reason out the drug's major therapeutic effects and applications, contraindications, and clinically important, mechanism-based adverse effects.
   - The student identifies clinically relevant, idiosyncratic adverse effects of commonly used drugs.

3) **The student describes proper techniques for preparing and administering vaccines, as well as explains common adverse effects associated with vaccine administration.**
   - The student displays understanding of the basic immunologic concepts underlying immunization.
   - The student recognizes the importance of:
     1) Using a new, sterile syringe and needle for each patient.
     2) Only using diluents provided or recommended by the manufacturer.
     3) Not mixing vaccines in the same syringe, unless recommended by the manufacturer.
     4) Using recommended sites and routes of administration for individual vaccines and noting vaccination sites in patient records.
     5) Administering vaccines within an appropriate time frame after reconstitution.
   - The student demonstrates the ability to identify and explain potential adverse reactions to vaccines, including, but not limited to, transient lethargy, low grade fever, vomiting, diarrhea, anaphylaxis, local inflammation at the injection site, granulomas, and vaccination-site sarcomas.
   - The student demonstrates the ability to distinguish clinically significant adverse reactions to vaccination and recognizes the urgent need for an appropriate response, including the immediate notification of a supervisor.

4) **The student accurately calculates drug doses and dosages, correctly using weights and measures.**
   - The student demonstrates understanding of relevant systems of weights and measures, including metric, apothecary and household systems, and describes their appropriate uses in the clinical setting.

Assessing Essential Skills of Veterinary Technology Students, Third Edition. Edited by Laurie J. Buell, Lisa E. Schenkel and Sabrina Timperman.
© 2017 John Wiley & Sons, Inc. Published 2017 by John Wiley & Sons, Inc.
Companion website: www.wiley.com/go/buell/skills

- The student accurately performs unit conversions, including but not limited to:
  1) Conversions between systems of measurement, such as pounds to kilograms.
  2) Conversions within systems of measurement, as in milliliters to liters.
- The student correctly calculates drug doses.
- The student accurately identifies and correctly uses the supplied dosage strength (e.g., mg/ml, mg/tab) to convert from units of dose (e.g., mg, mEq) to units for administration (e.g., tablets, ml).
- The student correctly measures doses, accurately reading calibrations on syringe barrels and droppers.

5) **The student demonstrates knowledge of appropriate routes and methods of administration for commonly used drugs. If more than one administration route and/or method is commonly used for a drug, the student displays knowledge of the correct clinical indications for each.**
   - The student demonstrates understanding of comparative rates of absorption and onsets of effect of various administration routes.
   - The student shows knowledge of drug types that should not be given subcutaneously or intramuscularly (e.g., agents that are extremely acidic or alkaline, vesicants, etc.).
   - The student displays knowledge of drugs that should not be administered intravenously (e.g., any drug not labeled for IV administration, repository preparations, suspensions or solutions with any sign of precipitation, etc.).
   - In selecting an appropriate route and method of drug administration, the student demonstrates the ability to consider the individual patient, the veterinarian's instructions and the prescribed drug to achieve the greatest therapeutic response while minimizing potential adverse responses. For example, the student considers individual patient status, correctly explaining that oral administration generally is contraindicated in a vomiting or dyspneic animal.

6) **The student explains the proper administration of drugs by prescribed routes, including common enteral and parenteral routes, at prescribed dosage intervals, describing safe and effective techniques.**
   - The student correctly describes commonly used enteral and parenteral administration routes.
   - The student describes proper technique for administering oral medications. The student demonstrates understanding of how to avoid complications such as esophageal stricture by administering an appropriate volume of water by mouth, following administration of oral tablets and capsules.
   - The student explains correct technique for administering drugs parenterally. The student identifies appropriate muscles for IM drug administration. The student identifies appropriate veins for IV drug administration. The student identifies appropriate sites for SC drug administration.

7) **The student displays knowledge of how to carefully monitor patients for therapeutic responses and adverse reactions to drugs.**
   - The student properly defines the terms "therapeutic response, adverse reaction, and side effect."
   - The student demonstrates the basic ability to recognize therapeutic effects of drugs and to distinguish them from adverse effects of drugs.

8) **The student demonstrates the ability to accurately enter all information pertaining to drug and/or vaccine administration in patients' medical records.**
   - The student displays the ability to precisely record information in the patient's record, including, but not limited to, the name of the drug, the dose administered, the route of administration, the site of administration, and when and by whom the medication or vaccine was administered.
   - The student uses correct drug names and properly uses veterinary abbreviations, where appropriate.

9) **The student displays knowledge of DEA regulations regarding scheduled (controlled) substances.**
   - The student correctly defines the terms "controlled or scheduled" drug. The student demonstrates practical understanding of the classification of controlled drugs into five schedules. The student accurately identifies common controlled drugs used therapeutically in practice and correctly classifies them as to Schedule (II–V) (Title 21 Code of Federal Regulations, 2016).
   - The student demonstrates knowledge and appreciates the importance of compliance with all federal and state regulations governing the purchase, storage, administration, dispensing, labeling, inventorying, and disposing of scheduled drugs.
   - The student describes the proper disposal of unused or expired controlled substances, in accordance with state and federal regulations.
   - The student completes a controlled substance inventory log, accurately recording each use in the controlled substance inventory log and in the patient's medical record. (The student records both the amount drawn up and the amount administered, when these quantities differ.)

10) **The student demonstrates knowledge of all state and federal regulations applicable to the purchase, storage, handling, dispensing, administration, disposal, and inventorying of drugs, biologics, pesticides, insecticides, and hazardous wastes derived from these substances.**
    - The student displays proficiency in accurately identifying and differentiating drugs, biologics, pesticides, insecticides, and hazardous waste.
    - The student demonstrates practical knowledge of state and federal regulations pertaining to these substances. This includes the roles of the Food and Drug Administration (FDA) in overseeing drug evaluation, approval and marketing, the United States Department of Agriculture (USDA) in regulating biologics (including vaccines, antitoxins, etc.), and the Drug Enforcement Agency (DEA) in enforcing federal laws and rules pertaining to controlled drugs.
    - The student demonstrates knowledge of potential safety concerns when working with and around pharmaceutical agents, biologics, insecticides, pesticides, and hazardous wastes derived from these agents.
    - The student displays appreciation of the importance of precisely following manufacturers' recommendations for the proper handling, storage, administration and disposal of pharmaceutical agents, biologics, insecticides, and pesticides

11) **The student demonstrates knowledge of how to properly prepare medications for administration.**
    - The student accurately reads drug labels, displaying knowledge of proprietary and non-proprietary drug names and dosage strengths. The student shows knowledge of how to select the correct (prescribed) drug and dosage strength. The student demonstrates understanding of the importance of carefully checking the label at least three times.
    - The student recognizes the need to check all drug containers for cracks, foreign matter, precipitation, color changes, expiration dates, reconstitution dates, and so on.
    - The student displays appreciation of the need to wash their hands prior to handling injectable agents and maintains aseptic technique, when appropriate.
    - The student demonstrates knowledge of how to select or prepare drugs in the prescribed form, correctly reconstituting drugs to desired dosage strengths when appropriate.

- The student selects appropriate equipment for drug administration, including:
  1) Choosing syringe size based on the volume of the dose and/or type (or dosage concentration) of drug. For example, using a 1 cc (tuberculin) syringe for a volume of 0.25 cc or using a U-100 insulin syringe for U-100 insulin.
  2) Choosing a needle gauge based on the quantity and type of fluid, administration route, and size, species, and age of the animal.

2.2 Pharmacy Essentials of Drug Dispensing

12) **The student displays the ability to properly prepare and dispense prescribed drugs to clients.**
    - The student demonstrates knowledge of the names of commonly used agents.
    - The student displays knowledge of veterinary terminology and abbreviations used in medication orders and prescriptions.
    - The student accurately performs appropriate dosage calculations, correctly using weights and measures.
    - The student demonstrates the ability to properly prepare drugs in the prescribed form, dose, dosage strength, and number of doses.

13) **The student demonstrates knowledge of the differences between prescription and over-the-counter drugs and abides by all laws and regulations applicable to each.**
    - The student demonstrates understanding of the concept that no drug is free of risks, and that all drugs are associated with potential hazardous or undesirable effects.
    - The student displays knowledge that prescription (legend) drugs are considered by the Food and Drug Administration (FDA) to be unsafe for use, except under the supervision of a veterinarian, physician or other practitioner licensed to prescribe drugs. The student demonstrates knowledge of over-the-counter (OTC) drugs as those that do not require the supervision of a licensed practitioner to be used and do not require a prescription to be purchased.
    - The student shows knowledge of FDA labeling, including (but not limited to) approved indications, contraindications, warnings, precautions, adverse reactions, dosage and administration.
    - The student demonstrates knowledge of the Animal Medicinal Drug Use Clarification Act (AMDUCA), and its provisions and requirements for extra-label drug use in animals (Food and Drug Administration, 2014).

14) **The student displays the ability to provide clients with appropriate, complete and accurate information when dispensing drugs.**
   - The student demonstrates adequate knowledge of commonly used therapeutic agents, including their proper handling, storage, administration, and therapeutic indications. The student demonstrates awareness of common adverse drug reactions and drug interactions.
   - The student displays the ability to communicate necessary drug information to clients in a manner that maximizes client understanding, compliance with prescribed therapy and safety for both the client and the patient.

15) **The student labels medications correctly and legibly, with proper directions to the client.**
   - The student lists complete, required information on prescription drug labels, including: the name, address and phone number of the veterinarian; the client's name, address and phone number, identification of the animal, species, number of animals (if treating a group, herd or flock); the date of treatment, prescribing or dispensing of the drug, the established name of the drug (active ingredient), the unit strength, dose, dosage frequency and duration, the route of administration, the quantity to be dispensed, the expiration date, precautionary information, and the number of refills, if any (American Veterinary Medical Association, 2015).
   - For food-producing animals, the student shows awareness that slaughter-withdrawal and/or milk-withholding times must be included, if applicable.
   - The student demonstrates understanding that state law and other regulations may require more or other information than listed before.
   - The student displays knowledge of labelling information required for extra-label use of drugs (Food and Drug Administration, 2014).

References

American Veterinary Medical Association. (2015). *Guidelines for Veterinary Prescription Drugs*. Retrieved May 11, 2016, from American Veterinary Medical Association: www.avma.org/KB/Policies/Pages/Guidelines-for-Veterinary-Prescription-Drugs.aspx (accessed September 14, 2016).

Food and Drug Administration. (2014, December 9). *Animal Medicinal Drug Use Clarification Act of 1994*. Retrieved May 10, 2016, from U.S. Food and Drug Administration: www.fda.gov/AnimalVeterinary/GuidanceComplianceEnforcement/ActsRulesRegulations/ucm085377.htm (accessed September 14, 2016)

Title 21 Code of Federal Regulations. (2016, February). *Controlled Substance Schedules*. Retrieved May 11, 2016, from Drug Enforcement Administration Office of Diversion Control: www.deadiversion.usdoj.gov/schedules/index.html.

3

Medical Nursing

Deirdre Douglas, Laurie J. Buell and Lisa E. Schenkel

3.1 Assessment of the Veterinary Patient

1) **The student displays the ability to effectively acquire subjective and objective information that permits accurate assessment of the patient's status.**
   - The student's actions show that they consider safety of personnel and patients to be of paramount importance in patient assessment.
   - The student is careful to thoroughly wash their hands between handling animals, before donning sterile gloves and after contact with body fluids or tissues.
   - The student successfully obtains accurate patient data and makes correct notations in the animal's medical record.

2) **The student displays knowledge of common domestic animal species and breeds.**
   - The student shows the ability to recognize common domestic animals and differentiate various breeds.
   - The student displays the ability to identify the sex of common domestic species.

3) **The student demonstrates the ability to explain and use common methods of animal identification.**
   - The student displays appreciation of the importance of properly identifying the patient upon admission to the facility and prior to every treatment.
   - The student shows knowledge that patient identification includes confirmation of the patient's name, age, sex, reproductive status, vaccine status, medical history (including reason for hospitalization), and pertinent behavioral information, for example, "will bite."
   - The student displays knowledge of how to properly label and use all appropriate facility techniques, such as neck bands and cage cards, to identify patients.

- The student demonstrates knowledge of microchips, including implantation techniques, use of handheld scanners, and the availability of different types of microchips.
- The student shows awareness of the use of tattoos as identification and common sites utilized.
- The student demonstrates knowledge of identification techniques for large animals, such as ear tagging, branding, and electronic identification.
- The student displays the ability to explain the advantages and disadvantages of common identification procedures.

4) **The student utilizes appropriate techniques when restraining cats and dogs for procedures.**
   - The student accurately assesses the patient's temperament.
   - The student utilizes appropriate restraint techniques when needed, based on species, size, temperament, medical status, and procedure to be performed.
   - The student restrains dogs and cats in a manner that promotes calmness and avoids stress and injury.

5) **The student effectively, safely, and properly encages and removes small animals from cages.**
   - The student approaches the cage carefully, accurately assesses the animal's temperament based on its behavior, and safely removes and encages the animal.
   - The student avoids stressing the animal, applying only appropriate restraint techniques as needed.

6) **The student effectively, safely, and correctly affixes muzzles on dogs.**
   - The student displays familiarity with different muzzle types, including basket muzzles, brachycephalic-specific muzzles, and rope or gauze.
   - The student appropriately restrains and safely applies muzzles to dogs.

Assessing Essential Skills of Veterinary Technology Students, Third Edition. Edited by Laurie J. Buell, Lisa E. Schenkel and Sabrina Timperman.
© 2017 John Wiley & Sons, Inc. Published 2017 by John Wiley & Sons, Inc.
Companion website: www.wiley.com/go/buell/skills

7) **The student effectively, safely, and correctly affixes Elizabethan collars.**
   - The student selects an Elizabethan collar (E-collar) of an appropriate size based on the animal's size, condition, and procedure.
   - The student effectively restrains the animal and securely affixes the E-collar on the animal.

8) **The student participates in and can explain how to effectively and correctly employ a restraint pole and other restraint aids.**
   - The student demonstrates knowledge of how to correctly use a restraint pole.
   - The student displays knowledge of how to correctly and appropriately use other restraint aides, such as towels and gloves.

9) **The student effectively, safely, and securely halters, ties, and leads horses.**
   - The student demonstrates awareness of equine behavior relevant to handling and restraint.
   - The student properly approaches the horse based on correct assessment of the horse's temperament.
   - Using appropriate restraint technique, the student properly applies a halter and lead rope.
   - The student demonstrates proper use of the lead rope to safely guide the horse.
   - The student displays understanding of when and how to properly use tying as a restraint technique for a horse.

10) **The student effectively, safely, and correctly restrains birds.**
   - The student demonstrates knowledge of the differences in avian species and of species-related restraint considerations. For example, claws are more likely to be of concern with raptors, while beaks are more likely to be of concern with psittacines.
   - The student shows understanding of the importance of minimizing stress in all avian species and never applying pressure across the thoracic area.
   - The student properly restrains birds, approaching them slowly and using appropriate technique based on species.

11) **The student participates in effectively, safely, and correctly implementing a twitch for equine restraint.**
   - The student demonstrates knowledge of proper placement of the twitch on the upper lip, avoiding the delicate inner surface.
   - The student displays knowledge of the correct manner of applying and twisting the twitch.
   - The student shows understanding of the importance of periodically loosening, tightening, and replacing the twitch.

12) **The student effectively, safely, and correctly implements bovine tail restraint.**
   - The student properly approaches the cow while it is positioned in a stanchion.
   - The student slowly lifts the tail using proper technique.
   - The student applies the appropriate amount of pressure to distract the cow's attention and lowers the tail slowly when the procedure is finished.

13) **The student effectively, safely, and correctly affixes halters to cattle.**
   - The student properly approaches cattle in a chute or stanchion from the side.
   - The student applies the halter in a manner that minimizes the chance of injury.

14) **The student participates in the safe and effective use of a cattle chute.**
   - The student displays knowledge of different chute configurations and their appropriate applications.
   - The student demonstrates knowledge of how to safely direct cattle into a chute.

15) **The student demonstrates the ability to acquire an accurate and thorough patient history.**
   - The student displays understanding of how to obtain all required information, including but not limited to, the presenting concern, past medical history, current medications, vaccine status, recent boarding, grooming or travel, reproductive status, and exposure to other animals.
   - The student shows understanding of how to phrase questions appropriately and avoid leading questions.
   - The student displays the ability to legibly and accurately record the history in a systematic, logical sequence, including all available dates.

16) **The student displays competence in safely and accurately determining and recording the temperature of the dog, cat, horse, and cow.**
   - The student shows knowledge of different thermometer types and their appropriate uses.
   - The student ensures the patient is appropriately restrained.
   - The student utilizes correct gentle technique, accurately reads the temperature, and records it in the patient's medical record.
   - The student cleans the patient and the thermometer appropriately.

17) **The student displays competence in safely and accurately determining and recording the pulse of the dog, cat, horse, and cow.**
   - The student recognizes multiple sites for obtaining the pulse and utilizes the appropriate site based on species and patient.

- The student palpates the pulse effectively and is able to recognize abnormalities.
- The student counts the pulse accurately and records the pulse in the patient's medical record.

18) **The student displays competence in safely and accurately determining and recording the respiratory rate of the dog, cat, horse, and cow.**
    - The student ensures that the patient is in a relaxed and comfortable position.
    - The student accurately counts the respiratory rate and discerns respiratory effort.
    - The student accurately records the respiratory rate and effort in the patient's medical record.

19) **The student displays competence in safely and accurately ausculting heart and lung sounds in the dog, cat, horse, and cow.**
    - The student ensures that the animal is appropriately restrained.
    - The student uses proper auscultation techniques based on species.
    - The student auscults multiple appropriate areas on both sides of the thorax to evaluate heart sounds.
    - The student auscults multiple appropriate areas on both sides of the thorax to evaluate lung sounds.
    - The student recognizes the need to palpate pulses while ausculting and demonstrates the ability to do so correctly.
    - The student correctly differentiates between normal and abnormal heart sounds and rhythms.
    - The student correctly distinguishes between normal and abnormal respiratory sounds, patterns, and effort.

20) **The student correctly obtains samples for diagnostic analysis, including blood, urine, feces, and specimens for cytology.**
    - The student properly selects and prepares, in advance, all necessary equipment and supplies.
    - The student correctly collects and stores fecal samples.
    - For ear cytology, the student properly obtains ear samples for cytology and culture and antimicrobial susceptibility testing prior to cleaning and/or treatment.
    - For vaginal cytology, the student properly prepares the external vaginal/vulvar area and obtains a vaginal sample.

21) **The student correctly performs venipuncture of the feline and canine cephalic vein.**
    - The student displays knowledge of the pertinent anatomy of the forelimb of cats and dogs.
    - The student considers the patient's species, breed, and medical condition when selecting the venipuncture site.

- The student selects the appropriate equipment and supplies, based on the test required, and prepares them in advance of performing venipuncture.
- The student makes certain that the dog and cat are properly restrained and the venipuncture site is correctly prepared.
- The student performs cephalic venipuncture using correct technique.
- The student aspirates an adequate and appropriate volume of blood into the syringe.
- The student makes certain that proper pressure is applied to the puncture site for an adequate time after the needle is withdrawn.

22) **The student correctly performs venipuncture of the feline, canine, equine, and ruminant jugular vein.**
    - The student displays knowledge of the pertinent anatomical structures in the neck of cats, dogs, horses and ruminants.
    - The student considers the patient's species, breed, and medical condition when selecting the venipuncture site.
    - The student selects the appropriate equipment and supplies based on the test required and prepares them in advance of performing venipuncture.
    - The student makes certain that the patient is properly restrained and the venipuncture site is correctly prepared.
    - The student performs jugular venipuncture using correct technique.
    - The student collects an adequate and appropriate volume of blood.
    - The student makes certain that proper pressure is applied to the puncture site for an adequate time after the needle is withdrawn.

23) **The student correctly performs venipuncture of the canine and feline saphenous vein.**
    - The student displays knowledge of the pertinent anatomy of the hindlimb in dogs and cats.
    - The student considers the patient's species, breed, and medical condition when selecting the venipuncture site.
    - The student selects the appropriate equipment and supplies based on the test required and prepares them in advance of performing venipuncture.
    - The student makes certain that the patient is properly restrained and the venipuncture site is correctly prepared.
    - The student performs saphenous venipuncture using correct technique.
    - The student collects an adequate and appropriate volume of blood.

- The student makes certain that proper pressure is applied to the puncture site for an adequate time after the needle is withdrawn.

24) **The student participates in obtaining a urine sample by urethral catheterization of the male dog.**
    - The student displays knowledge of the pertinent urinary tract anatomy in the dog.
    - The student demonstrates understanding of the need to gently and aseptically place urinary catheters to decrease risks of trauma and catheter-associated urinary tract infections.
    - The student prepares all sterile equipment in advance, including appropriately-sized urinary catheters, lubricant, gloves, syringes, and sample containers.
    - The student demonstrates knowledge of how to appropriately restrain the animal in a position that enables grasping the prepuce.
    - The student displays knowledge of how to aseptically prepare the patient.
    - The student participates in the catheterization of the urethra and collection of the urine sample, using correct technique.

25) **The student correctly obtains a voided urine sample from the dog and cat.**
    - The student displays understanding of the importance of using the correct technique to obtain a urine sample.
    - To collect voided urine from the dog, the student properly cleans the prepuce or vulva with antiseptic solution.
    - The student successfully catches a midstream sample into a clean/sterile container, withdrawing the container prior to end of urination.
    - To collect voided urine from the cat, the student places the litter box in the cage with no litter or with non-absorbent material. The student properly collects the urine from the litter box.

26) **The student participates in correctly performing cystocentesis in the dog or cat.**
    - The student displays knowledge of the pertinent abdominal anatomy of the dog and cat.
    - The student shows awareness of potential complications caused by improper cystocentesis, such as trauma to the urinary bladder and/or abdominal tissues, enterocentesis and hemorrhage due to accidental puncture of the aorta.
    - The student displays awareness that ultrasound-guided cystocentesis may help to minimize the risk of complications.
    - The student demonstrates understanding of how to restrain the animal in the proper position.
    - The student displays knowledge of how to aseptically prepare the patient for cystocentesis.

- The student explains the proper procedure for performing cystocentesis in small animals.
- The student appropriately participates in the collection of a urine sample via cystocentesis.
- The student understands the need to give the patient the opportunity to urinate after cystocentesis.

27) **The student displays knowledge of how to properly prepare, handle, and store diagnostic samples for shipment.**
    - The student shows knowledge of how to identify and use appropriate tubes, containers and slides for shipping hematological, serological, urine, fluid, and tissue samples.
    - The student demonstrates understanding of the importance of collecting sterile samples in sealed, sterile containers, and displays the ability to correctly label containers.
    - The student displays understanding of the importance of accurately completing laboratory forms and properly packaging samples.
    - The student demonstrates the ability to accurately complete laboratory forms and properly package samples.

3.2 Nursing Care of the Veterinary Patient

3.2.1 Husbandry of Common Domestic Species

Deirdre Douglas, Lisa E. Schenkel, Laurie J. Buell and Sabrina Timperman

28) **The student displays knowledge of how to properly therapeutically bathe, groom, and dip small animals.**
    - The student shows knowledge of various types of therapeutic shampoos and dips, including indications for use.
    - The student explains how to properly bathe and apply chemical dips to small animals.
    - The student demonstrates understanding of the importance of protecting the patient's eyes from chemical injury, preventing excess water from entering the external ear canal, and avoiding chemical and thermal injury.
    - The student displays knowledge of the potential toxic effects of chemical dips and can explain correct dilution techniques.
    - The student shows knowledge of how to correctly utilize protective gear when applying chemical dips and shampoos.
    - The student describes how to appropriately warm and dry animals.
    - The student explains how to properly utilize brushes and combs, as well as remove matted fur.

- The student explains the importance of checking the ambient temperature and monitoring for signs of hyper- and/or hypothermia, as well as for adverse reactions.

29) **The student correctly trims nails of dogs and cats.**
   - The student shows knowledge of the fact that dogs and cats have claws (rather than nails).
   - The student displays knowledge of claw anatomy in dogs and cats.
   - The student properly trims the claws of dogs and cats using the correct tools and techniques.
   - The student displays knowledge of the proper use of cauterizing agents/hemostatic techniques, and correctly utilizes them when needed.

30) **The student properly applies tail and leg wraps to horses.**
   - The student identifies relevant anatomical structures and anticipates potential problem areas.
   - The student displays understanding of indications for leg and tail wraps.
   - The student properly restrains the patient for wrap application.
   - The student cleans/washes and dries the foot and hoof areas before applying leg wraps.
   - The student properly applies various tail wraps, including gauze, bandage material and commercially available tail bags.

31) **The student correctly expresses canine anal sacs.**
   - The student accurately identifies the position of anal sacs and ducts.
   - The student demonstrates understanding of potential complications of the procedure, including anal sac rupture and rectal tearing.
   - The student correctly inserts a gloved, lubricated finger into the rectum and expresses the anal sacs, using appropriate pressure. The student thoroughly cleans the perianal area.
   - The student correctly distinguishes normal from abnormal anal sac secretions.

32) **The student properly cleans ears and administers otic medications in dogs and cats.**
   - The student demonstrates knowledge of the anatomy of the external ear canal.
   - The student demonstrates understanding of the importance of physical or chemical restraint due to the sensitivity of inflamed ears.
   - The student correctly administers ear flushes and/or properly applies appropriate ear cleaning solutions. The student uses correct technique for cleaning ears.
   - The student correctly applies appropriate ear medications.
   - The student demonstrates proper technique for medicating ears to the owner and communicates the importance of compliance.

33) **The student effectively carries out sanitation procedures for animal holding and housing areas.**
   - The student displays knowledge of infectious disease transmission, including direct and indirect routes.
   - The student demonstrates understanding of the importance of sanitation and its significance in disease prevention/transmission as well as reducing patient stress.
   - The student shows understanding of the purpose of isolation areas, including the importance of following strict sanitation and disinfection procedures in isolation areas as well as the importance of preventing animals with no infectious disease from occupying isolation areas.
   - The student effectively implements sanitation procedures.
   - The student shows knowledge of the efficacies, relative advantages and potential disadvantages/toxicities of various disinfectants in use in veterinary facilities.
   - The student appropriately uses various disinfectants.

34) **The student demonstrates knowledge of various methods of permanent identification in common domestic species.**
   - The student demonstrates knowledge of appropriate uses and relative advantages and disadvantages of various methods of identifying large domestic animals, such as tattooing, ear tagging, branding, and electronic methods.
   - The student demonstrates knowledge of permanent identification methods in small animals, such as microchipping.

35) **The student demonstrates knowledge of breeding and reproduction procedures.**
   - The student demonstrates knowledge of the estrous cycle in common domestic species and recognizes signs of each stage. The student shows understanding of the care of the female in estrus and is able to explain proper care to the owner.
   - The student demonstrates knowledge of the mating behavior of common domestic species.
   - The student demonstrates knowledge of the gestation periods of common domestic species. The student explains how to provide appropriate care for the pregnant female.
   - The student shows knowledge of the signs of approaching parturition. The student demonstrates knowledge of signs and behaviors associated with stages of labor and birth.
   - The student explains how to assist in normal delivery and care of newborns.

36) **The student demonstrates understanding of the proper nursing care of neonates and its role in enhancing wellness and reducing risk of disease, injury, and stress.**
   - The student demonstrates knowledge of requirements for: maintaining appropriate ambient temperature; hydration; importance of colostrum; proper nutrition and food types; quantity and frequency of feeding; elimination; correct hygiene; proper housing; and socialization.
   - The student displays knowledge of common neonatal problems, including dehydration, hypothermia, hypoglycemia, vomiting, diarrhea, elimination difficulties, and anorexia.
   - The student shows understanding of proper nursing care for the neonatal problems listed here.
   - The student shows the ability to communicate appropriate instructions for neonatal care to owners.

3.2.2 Nutrition of Common Domestic Species

Deirdre Douglas, Lisa E. Schenkel, Sabrina Timperman and Laurie J. Buell

37) **For the dog, cat, horse, and cow, the student demonstrates knowledge of nutritional requirements for each stage of life.**
   - The student shows understanding of appropriate (and inappropriate) dietary components for optimal health in various life stages.
   - The student demonstrates the ability to explain nutritional recommendations for various life stages to owners and reinforce owner compliance.

38) **The student demonstrates understanding of the role of nutrients and nutrition in disease states and shows familiarity with therapeutic diets.**
   - The student displays understanding of the importance of providing adequate and appropriate nutrition for patients.
   - The student shows understanding of enteral and parenteral routes of nutritional support and the appropriate indications for each.
   - The student demonstrates knowledge of specific nutritional requirements in common disease states.
   - The student displays understanding of the appropriate uses of therapeutic regimens (e.g., prescription diets) in order to enhance recovery and manage chronic diseases.
   - The student is able to explain to owners the need for special or therapeutic diets to enhance recovery and manage chronic diseases, and to reinforce owner compliance.

39) **The student demonstrates current knowledge of commonly used nutritional supplements and food additives, including their potential benefits and toxic effects.**
   - The student demonstrates awareness of the potential benefits of use of substances classified as nutritional supplements, such as vitamins, minerals, herbs, botanicals, amino acids, and others.
   - The student demonstrates understanding of the fact that the FDA does not have authority to require research and FDA approval prior to marketing nutritional supplements. Therefore, manufacturers of nutritional supplements may legally make claims about conditions associated with natural states without FDA approval, even though the efficacy and potential adverse effects have not been identified in controlled studies. In addition, the student shows awareness of the fact that the FDA cannot require removal of nutritional supplements from the market unless the FDA proves significant risk of illness or injury.
   - The student demonstrates awareness of the fact that any substance, including herbal and/or "all-natural" substances, are potentially associated with toxicities at some dose.
   - The student shows understanding of the fact that there may be serious interactions between drugs and nutritional supplements.

40) **The student displays knowledge of and is able to identify common poisonous plants.**
   - The student identifies common poisonous plants including, but not limited to, *Euphorbia* spp. (poinsettia), *Hydrangea* spp., *Ilex* spp. (holly), *Narcissus* spp. (daffodil), *Nerium* spp. (oleander), *Philodendron* spp., *Phoradendron* spp. (mistletoe), *Toxicodendron* spp. (poison ivy, poison oak), lilies, onions, moldy sweet clover, and so on.
   - The student shows knowledge of toxic effects caused by common poisonous plants.

41) **The student demonstrates knowledge of and is able to identify common substances that produce toxic effects when ingested.**
   - The student displays familiarity with toxicities associated with such substances as commonly used drugs, insecticides (including, but not limited to, organophosphates, limonene, and other citrus oil extracts, etc.), chocolate, caffeine, ethylene glycol, fertilizers, household cleaning products, xylitol, and so on.

42) **The student demonstrates the ability to develop and effectively communicate hospital nutritional protocols.**
   - The student displays the ability to utilize their knowledge of nutritional requirements to create appropriate nutritional protocols for hospitalized patients.

- The student shows the ability to effectively communicate nutritional protocols to veterinary staff members in order to ensure continuity of care.

3.2.3 Therapeutics for Common Domestic Species

Lisa E. Schenkel, Laurie J. Buell, Sabrina Timperman, Nicole VanSant and Deirdre Douglas

43) **In light of the veterinarian's directions and the individual patient's characteristics and physical status, the student demonstrates the ability to administer injectable medications in a manner that maximally enhances health benefits for the patient.**
   - The student shows knowledge of appropriate routes of injection for commonly used medications as well as differences among parenteral administration routes regarding relative rates of absorption, onset of effect, and duration of effect. The student displays knowledge of potential complications associated with common parenteral administration routes.
   - The student demonstrates appreciation of the importance of accurately identifying and selecting correct medications and of checking the label at least three times to assure selection of the correct drug, dosage concentration, administration route, and so on.
   - The student displays understanding of the importance of checking the bottle for cracks, expiration dates, reconstitution dates, foreign matter, color changes, precipitation, and so on.
   - The student shows knowledge of how to use correct aseptic technique.

44) **The student properly administers subcutaneous injections to dogs, cats, and ruminants.**
   - The student demonstrates the ability to determine proper injection sites in common domestic species.
   - The student appropriately prepares the site for injection.
   - The student selects the appropriate size/gauge syringe and needle.
   - The student properly holds the syringe and inserts the needle at the correct angle and depth.
   - The student aspirates the syringe to check for blood and/or improper placement.
   - The student administers the correct dose of medication, withdraws the needle and gently massages the injection site.
   - The student properly disposes of the syringe and needle.

45) **The student properly administers intramuscular injections to dogs, cats, and horses.**
   - The student demonstrates the ability to determine proper injection sites in common domestic species.
   - The student appropriately prepares the site for injection.
   - The student selects the appropriate size/gauge syringe and needle.
   - The student properly holds the syringe and inserts the needle at the correct angle and depth.
   - The student aspirates the syringe to check for blood and/or improper placement.
   - The student administers the correct dose of medication, withdraws the needle and gently massages the injection site.
   - The student properly disposes of the syringe and needle.

46) **The student correctly administers direct-bolus, intravenous injections to dogs, cats, ruminants, and horses.**
   - The student demonstrates the ability to identify proper injection sites in common domestic species.
   - The student accurately palpates and isolates the vein for injection.
   - The student appropriately prepares the site for injection, using an assistant or a tourniquet to "raise" and stabilize the vein.
   - The student properly holds the syringe and inserts the needle into the vein at the correct angle, aspirating the syringe to check for blood in the hub.
   - When administering medications with a butterfly catheter, the student correctly holds the catheter and inserts the needle into the vein at a correct angle, allowing the blood to fill the tubing.
   - The student removes the tourniquet or has the assistant release pressure on the vein at the appropriate time.
   - The student administers a correct dose of medication, at an appropriate administration rate (time interval), while making certain that the needle is properly stabilized in the vein and that the entire dose is given intravenously.
   - When using a butterfly catheter, the student appropriately flushes the catheter following the injection of medication.
   - The student withdraws the needle and applies appropriate pressure to the venipuncture site to stop bleeding.

47) **The student considers the individual patient's characteristics and physical status when administering non-injectable medications in order to provide maximal benefits with minimal risk and stress to the patient.**
   - The student displays knowledge of various enteral administration routes and of potential complications associated with each.

- The student demonstrates appreciation of the importance of accurately identifying and selecting correct medications and of checking the label at least three times to assure selection of the correct drug, dosage concentration, administration route, and so on.
- The student displays understanding of the importance of checking the bottle for cracks, expiration dates, reconstitution dates, foreign matter, color changes, precipitation, and so on.

48) **The student demonstrates the ability to properly utilize a balling gun to administer medications to ruminants.**
   - The student appropriately restrains the animal and demonstrates awareness of safety protocols.
   - The student demonstrates proper use of the balling gun.
   - The student monitors the patient to be certain the medication is properly received.

49) **The student displays the ability to correctly utilize a dose syringe to administer medications to ruminants and horses.**
   - The student appropriately restrains the animal and demonstrates awareness of safety protocols.
   - The student demonstrates the ability to administer small volumes of liquid, using a dose syringe.
   - The student monitors the patient to be certain the medication is properly received.

50) **The student participates in the correct placement of a stomach tube in small animals.**
   - The student demonstrates awareness of potential complications of stomach tube placement in small animals.
   - The student displays knowledge of various types of stomach tubes, such as nasogastric and orogastric, and their appropriate indications.
   - The student describes how to select an appropriate size tube based on the patient's size.
   - The student explains proper techniques for stomach tube placement.
   - The student shows knowledge of how to check for proper stomach tube placement.

51) **The student properly hand-pills dogs and cats.**
   - The student understands contraindications to and potential complications of oral administration of medications.
   - The student employs proper technique for hand-pilling the dog, while maintaining safe restraint.
   - The student employs proper technique for hand-pilling the cat, while maintaining safe restraint.

- The student administers water via syringe following the oral administration of dry drugs to assist in the movement of the drug through the esophagus and into the stomach as well as to avoid esophageal injury/stricture.
- The student monitors the animal to make certain the medication was properly received.

52) **The student correctly administers topical and ophthalmic medications.**
   - The student describes precautions for handling and safety when administering topical and ophthalmic medications
   - For topical medications, the student clips and cleanses the affected area as needed.
   - Wearing gloves, the student applies the proper amount of topical medication.
   - To administer ophthalmic medications, the student properly restrains the animal's head and, keeping the head stable, opens the eyelid.
   - The student properly administers ocular drops/ointment, ensuring that the applicator tip does not touch the eye and remains sterile.
   - The student makes certain that the animal does not rub its eye with its paws or rub its eye against any object immediately post-treatment.
   - When necessary, the student applies an e-collar to prevent the animal from reaching the affected area.

53) **The student correctly performs ocular diagnostic tests, including the Schirmer tear test, fluorescein staining, and tonometry.**
   - The student demonstrates knowledge of keratoconjunctivitis sicca (KCS) and can explain the role of the Schirmer tear test in its diagnosis.
   - The student makes certain to perform the Schirmer tear test prior to any other procedures involving the eye.
   - The student properly holds and controls the animal's head. The student correctly performs the Schirmer tear test.
   - The student accurately measures the length of the strip from the notch to the wet/dry interface.
   - The student can differentiate between normal and abnormal results on the Schirmer tear test.
   - The student demonstrates understanding of the use of fluorescein staining to detect corneal ulceration or other damage to the corneal epithelium.
   - With the animal's head properly restrained, the student opens the lid and correctly applies fluorescein stain to the eye.
   - Using a cobalt blue light, the student examines the eye for signs of epithelial damage.
   - The student displays the ability to recognize the normal appearance of the corneal epithelium and

to distinguish signs of corneal epithelial damage as seen under cobalt blue light.

- The student demonstrates knowledge that tonometry is used to measure intraocular pressure.
- The student displays awareness that minimal restraint is essential for performing tonometry, because excessive restraint can falsely elevate intraocular pressure.
- The student demonstrates the ability to properly administer one drop of short-acting, local, ophthalmic anesthetic agent (e.g., proparacaine) onto each eye. The student correctly uses a tonometer to accurately measure intraocular pressure.
- The student correctly reads and records intraocular pressure.
- The student can distinguish between normal and abnormal intraocular pressures.

54) **The student participates in the proper administration of enemas.**
- The student demonstrates understanding of potential complications of administering enemas, such as damage to rectal mucosa, transmission of infection, and so on. The student shows awareness that enemas should be performed only when indicated, due to their potential risks.
- The student shows understanding of the advantages and potential adverse effects of different enema solutions.
- The student prepares all equipment in advance, making certain enema solutions are at or near body temperature.
- When administering enemas to cats, the student makes certain that a clean litter box is waiting in the cage.
- The student describes proper restraint of the animal.
- The student explains the proper procedure for administration of enemas.
- The student displays appreciation of the need to quickly move the animal to a run/cage or outdoors immediately after enema administration in order to allow bowel evacuation.
- The student shows appreciation of the importance of cleaning and drying the animal's hindquarters and placing the animal in a clean run/cage after bowel evacuation.

55) **The student correctly obtains and microscopically evaluates skin scrapings.**
- The student correctly identifies the lesion to be scraped. The student describes proper techniques for superficial and deep skin scrapings and the indications for each.
- The student properly performs the skin scraping.

- The student transfers collected hair and epithelial debris to a glass slide by scraping the material against the edge of the slide and, then, mixes the collected material with the mineral oil.
- The student microscopically examines and correctly evaluates the collected material, and appropriately records the results in the animal's medical record.

56) **The student properly administers fluids by the subcutaneous route.**
- The student demonstrates understanding of the pertinent anatomy.
- The student is able to differentiate types of fluids that may be administered subcutaneously from those that should not.
- The student displays understanding of how subcutaneous fluids are absorbed, the amount of fluid that can be safely administered by the subcutaneous route and potential complications associated with the subcutaneous administration of fluids.
- The student properly prepares all needed equipment in advance, including the correct fluid bag, the appropriate administration set and needle gauge, avoiding contamination. The student inspects the fluid bag for expiration date, integrity of sterile packaging, discoloration, cloudiness, and so on. If appropriate, the student pre-warms the fluids to body temperature.
- The student appropriately restrains the animal.
- The student properly identifies and prepares the administration site.
- Using correct technique, the student administers the correct volume of fluids at an appropriate flow rate, monitoring for patency of the administration set and the correct placement of the needle. The student clamps off the tubing and withdraws the needle, then applies pressure to injection site.
- The student displays the ability to explain and demonstrate to an owner how to properly and safely administer subcutaneous fluids, how they are absorbed, and their benefits to the animal. The student demonstrates the ability to properly educate clients as to the safe disposal of needles.

57) **The student properly places intravenous catheters into the cephalic and saphenous veins.**
- The student demonstrates knowledge of the pertinent anatomy, relative advantages and disadvantages of each site, and the potential complications associated with catheterization of each site.
- The student displays knowledge of the indications for use, benefits, and limitations of each catheter type.

- The student prepares, in advance, all necessary equipment, such as sterile gloves, scrub solution, alcohol, gauze pads, bandage material, tape, appropriate size and type of catheter, T-connector, or injection cap, saline or heparinized saline flushes, empty syringes, blood tubes, clippers, and so on.
- The student has the assistant appropriately position and restrain the animal.
- With gloved hands, the student aseptically prepares the site. The student correctly isolates, palpates, raises and stabilizes the vein. Wearing sterile gloves and maintaining aseptic technique, the student correctly and successfully places the catheter in the vein. The student verifies proper placement and patency of the catheter.
- The student properly secures the catheter with tape in a way that minimizes trauma to the vein.
- The student appropriately applies the bandage in a manner that secures placement of the catheter, permits access to the catheter for blood sampling, administration of fluids or medication; and minimizes discomfort to the patient.

58) **The student properly cares for and attentively monitors intravenous catheters.**

- The student displays knowledge of complications associated with indwelling intravenous catheters.
- When indicated, the student flushes indwelling catheters (e.g., with heparinized saline solution), checking their patency and integrity.
- At appropriate intervals, the student checks for signs of inflammation, infection, swelling or patient discomfort; the student also checks the bandage for slippage, moisture, cleanliness, or signs of patient discomfort.

59) **The student accurately calculates fluid infusion rates and explains how to monitor fluid administration to ensure correct administration rates.**

- The student defines the terms hydration deficit, maintenance requirements and ongoing losses and demonstrates understanding of the clinical implications of each.
- The student displays knowledge of various crystalloid solutions, including which are balanced versus non-balanced solutions and which are isotonic, hypotonic, or hypertonic. The student shows awareness of proper indications and major contraindications for various types of crystalloid solutions, as well as any special requirements for their administration.
- The student displays knowledge of various colloids, including natural and synthetic, their proper indications and any special requirements for their administration.

- The student accurately calculates fluid requirements, considering hydration deficits, maintenance requirements, and ongoing losses.
- The student accurately calculates appropriate fluid infusion rates.
- The student displays understanding of how to administer fluids at appropriate rates and how to monitor to ensure that the fluid is flowing freely at the correct rate.
- The student demonstrates knowledge of common additives, such as KCl solution, Vitamin B complex and 50% dextrose solution.
- The student shows understanding of the importance of correctly labeling fluid bags to indicate additives per liter bag of fluids.
- The student displays knowledge of common problems that can occur with fluid administration, such as a kink in the administration set, a clot in the catheter, a malfunction of the infusion pump, and so on, and explains how to correct them.

60) **The student demonstrates knowledge of how to correctly monitor and evaluate the hydration status of patients.**

- The student demonstrates knowledge of body fluid compartments. The student distinguishes classical signs associated with fluid losses from each body fluid compartment.
- The student explains how to evaluate patient hydration status qualitatively by assessment of skin turgor, moistness of mucous membranes, positioning of the eye within its socket, thoracic auscultation, pulse rate and strength, and patient demeanor. In animals receiving subcutaneous fluids, the student evaluates ventral or dependent anatomic areas to assess fluid absorption.
- The student describes how to evaluate patient hydration status quantitatively by accurate measurement of body weight (using same scale each time), PCV, plasma proteins, urine specific gravity (and urine output, if necessary).
- The student displays understanding of central venous pressure (CVP) and its role in assessing hydration status.
- The student demonstrates knowledge of how to recognize signs of overhydration by evaluation of lung sounds, heart rate, respiratory rate, conjunctiva, the presence of peripheral edema or serous nasal discharge, and/or increased urination.

61) **The student demonstrates familiarity with various fluid delivery systems.**

- The student shows knowledge of various fluid delivery systems, such as macrodrip and microdrip administration sets, volume control systems (Buretrol® sets), secondary administration sets and extension sets.

- The student demonstrates the ability to operate infusion pumps correctly.

62) **The student properly applies and removes bandages and splints.**
   - The student demonstrates understanding of the need to bandage wounds, fractures, catheter sites, and so on. The student demonstrates knowledge of indications for different bandage types.
   - The student displays knowledge of different types of primary bandaging materials, such as paraffin gauze, perforated film dressing, foam dressing and hydrocolloids, and their clinical application on the wound.
   - The student correctly applies bandages, including, but not limited to, the following steps: the student applies stirrups, selects appropriate primary, secondary, and tertiary layers and applies an appropriate protective layer.
   - The student demonstrates an understanding of appropriate uses of different types/sizes of splints and correctly applies them.
   - The student demonstrates knowledge of specialized bandages appropriate to specific situations, including, but not limited to, Robert Jones bandages, chest or abdominal bandages, Velpeau slings, and Ehmer slings.
   - The student explains appropriate bandage care and how to recognize and address complications.
   - The student correctly and safely removes bandages and splints.

63) **The student displays knowledge of appropriate care of wounds and abscesses.**
   - The student demonstrates knowledge of appropriate wound management and abscess care, including the immediate care of the wound or abscess; lavage and debridement; methods of wound closure and their appropriate uses, based on the individual wound.
   - The student demonstrates understanding of the appropriate uses of topical and systemic therapeutics for wounds and abscesses.

64) **The student demonstrates the ability to explain proper care of the recumbent patient.**
   - The student demonstrates understanding of basic requirements for care of recumbent patients, including, but not limited to, proper bedding, turning the patient to avoid hypostatic congestion and decubitus, passive range of motion (PROM) to reduce muscle atrophy and maintain joint mobility, monitoring of urine/stool output, TPR, nutritional requirements, and mental stimulation.
   - The student displays appreciation of the importance of keeping the recumbent patient clean and dry.

65) **The student participates in collecting and cross-match testing blood for transfusion.**
   - The student displays knowledge of canine and feline blood types.
   - The student shows understanding of the importance of crossmatch testing.
   - The student demonstrates knowledge of potential complications of incompatible blood transfusions.
   - The student correctly identifies and labels blood collection tubes for recipient and donor blood samples.
   - The student participates in properly performing crossmatch testing.
   - The student correctly identifies the presence or absence of agglutination. The student accurately interprets test results and correctly chooses an appropriate donor.

66) **The student demonstrates knowledge of how to properly stock and maintain an emergency crash cart.**
   - The student shows appreciation of the importance of preparing and maintaining an emergency crash cart.
   - The student displays knowledge of the essential components of a well-stocked, mobile emergency crash cart.
   - The student describes how to properly maintain a well-organized, mobile emergency crash cart.
   - The student demonstrates familiarity with all equipment needed to perform successful CPR, and explains how to regularly perform necessary equipment maintenance.
   - The student demonstrates awareness of the uses, indications, major contraindications, common adverse effects, and appropriate administration routes of commonly used emergency drugs.

67) **The student demonstrates competence in administering first aid and cardiopulmonary resuscitation (CPR).**
   - The student demonstrates knowledge of safety protocols for administering first aid to patients. For example, injured animals should be appropriately restrained because they may become aggressive due to fear and pain.
   - The student displays knowledge of how to safely transport an injured animal, demonstrating understanding of the importance of minimizing movement.
   - The student shows knowledge of the proper techniques for minimizing hemorrhage.
   - The student demonstrates knowledge of the proper techniques for stabilizing fractures.

- The student displays knowledge of how to prioritize patients for assessment by the veterinarian.
- The student demonstrates the ability to accurately identify patients most at risk for respiratory and/or cardiopulmonary arrest. The student shows knowledge of disease processes and/or drugs (including anesthetic and analgesic agents) that may predispose animals to respiratory and/or cardiopulmonary arrest.
- The student demonstrates appreciation of the importance of recognizing and treating abnormalities before arrest occurs (i.e., preventing arrest is better than treating arrest).
- The student shows understanding of the fact that preparedness and early recognition increase the chance of successful cardiopulmonary resuscitation (CPR).
- The student shows understanding of the importance of training and regularly practicing CPR with all available staff members.
- The student demonstrates knowledge of normal vital signs. The student recognizes normal cardiac rhythms and demonstrates the ability to differentiate normal from abnormal. The student recognizes normal respiratory rates, depths, and patterns and demonstrates the ability to differentiate normal from abnormal.
- The student displays understanding of the importance of closely monitoring vital signs in all patients at risk for respiratory and/or cardiopulmonary arrest. In patients under general anesthesia, the student shows understanding of the importance of closely observing vital signs and anesthetic monitoring equipment, as well as carefully and frequently evaluating respiratory function (adequacy of oxygenation and ventilation), circulatory function, and the degree of CNS depression (decreases in muscle tone and CNS reflexes).
- The student demonstrates knowledge of how to promptly recognize signs of impending cardiopulmonary arrest (CPA), including significant, abnormal changes in respiratory frequency, character (depth and/or pattern), or sound (agonal gasps); weak and/or significantly abnormal pulses; arrhythmias and/or changes in heart sounds; significant changes in body temperature and/or blood pressure; and/or abnormal mucous membrane color. In patients under general anesthesia, the student also shows knowledge of other indicators of impending arrest, including, but not limited to, significant abnormalities in SpO_2, pH, PaO_2, PvO_2, $ETCO_2$, and/or severe loss of muscle tone and CNS reflexes.
- The student exhibits knowledge of how to promptly recognize signs of cardiopulmonary arrest, including unconsciousness; absence of heart sounds and palpable pulses; absence of ventilatory efforts and breath sounds (agonal gasps may be heard); cyanotic, gray, or white mucous membranes; dilated pupils (within 1–2 minutes after arrest). The student demonstrates awareness that the veterinarian must be alerted immediately to signs of CPA.
- The student demonstrates knowledge of all components of CPR, including, but not limited to, the importance of team preparedness and communication, airway management, cardiovascular management, venous access, drug administration, and monitoring the effectiveness of CPR.
- The student shows understanding that the primary objective of basic life support (BLS) is to temporarily support the patient by administering artificial respirations (to oxygenate blood and remove CO_2) and administering chest compressions (to force adequate oxygenated blood into the coronary arteries to perfuse the myocardium and into the cerebral arteries to perfuse the brain). The student demonstrates knowledge of advanced life support, including commonly used drugs and recommended routes of administration for each (e.g., central venous catheter, intratracheal, intraosseous, and peripheral catheters); the role of fluid therapy; and electrical defibrillation.
- The student displays knowledge of the CPR guidelines contained in the 2012 RECOVER CPR initiative (Fletcher, et al., 2012).
  a) The student recognizes that high quality, uninterrupted chest compressions are the most important factor in successful CPR and should begin as soon as the arrest is recognized.
  b) The student demonstrates understanding of the thoracic and cardiac pump theories.
- The student properly performs external chest compressions, following the 2012 RECOVER guidelines for appropriate technique and rate (Fletcher, et al., 2012).
  a) The student correctly positions the animal for chest compressions.
  b) Based on the patient's chest conformation, the student correctly positions their hands and upper body to maximize the effectiveness of chest compressions.
  c) While performing chest compressions, the student keeps their arms straight and uses the upper body to compress the chest by one-third to one-half of its original width.
  d) The student displays understanding of the importance of two-minute cycles in basic life support and appropriately rotates positions with another team member in order to minimize fatigue and maximize the effectiveness of chest compressions.

e) The student demonstrates understanding of various methods of monitoring effectiveness of chest compressions, including, but not limited to, palpating pulses, capnography, and ECG monitoring.

- The student recognizes that the second priority in CPR is to secure an unobstructed airway, which usually is achieved by intubation with an endotracheal tube. (Tracheostomy tubes may be required in individual cases.) The student properly places endotracheal tubes. The student displays understanding of the importance of using suction, when necessary, to clear the oral cavity or ET tube of blood, mucus, foreign material, and so on.

- The student correctly uses the anesthetic machine or resuscitation (e.g., Ambu®) bag to deliver 100% oxygen to the patient. The student demonstrates understanding of the fact that, although delivery of 100% oxygen is ideal, when an oxygen source is unavailable, a resuscitation (e.g., Ambu®) bag may be used to deliver room air.

- The student properly administers positive-pressure ventilations, following the 2012 RECOVER guidelines for appropriate technique and rate (Fletcher, et al., 2012). The student displays knowledge of maximal inspiratory pressures as well as the potential adverse effects of exceeding them.

- The student demonstrates knowledge of the importance of capnography in assessing the effectiveness of chest compressions and in detecting the return of spontaneous circulation. The student displays the ability to accurately interpret capnography, relative to assessing chest compressions and detection of return of spontaneous circulation.

- The student displays knowledge of the importance of ECG monitoring in guiding advanced life support. The student evidences the ability to identify the dysrhythmias commonly associated with cardiopulmonary arrest.

- The student demonstrates understanding of the immediate need for venous access in CPR, providing that this does not require interruption of chest compressions.

- The student demonstrates knowledge of common drugs and IV fluid therapy used in CPR. The student shows familiarity with appropriate routes of administration for individual drugs, including IV, intratracheal, and/or intraosseous administration.

- The student shows knowledge of indications for use of electrical defibrillation as well as precautions necessary for its safe use.

- The student demonstrates understanding of the importance of close post-resuscitation monitoring and can explain how to properly assess patient status, such as level of consciousness and vital signs.

68) **The student correctly uses a resuscitation (e.g., Ambu®) bag.**
- The student properly uses a resuscitation (e.g., Ambu®) bag to deliver positive-pressure ventilations, using appropriate sizes for individual patients.

- The student properly connects the resuscitation (e.g., Ambu®) bag to a 100% oxygen source.

- In the ideal situation, the student keeps the bag connected at all times to an oxygen supply. However, when a 100% oxygen source is unavailable, the student demonstrates the ability to use a resuscitation (e.g., Ambu®) bag to deliver room air (21% oxygen).

69) **The student properly applies emergency splints and bandages.**
- The student recognizes indications for bandages or splints in emergency situations and demonstrates the ability to explain their benefits.

- The student selects an appropriate primary layer based on the wound type. The student selects the appropriate type of bandage.

- The student properly and quickly applies bandages in emergency situations, paying particular attention to location and pressure aspects of bandaging.

- The student explains proper bandage/splint care. The student describes how to recognize failed bandages/splints and how to take corrective measures.

3.3 Dental Procedures in Small Animals

Howard Gittelman

70) **In light of the patient's characteristics, species and condition, the student demonstrates the ability to accurately evaluate the patient's oral cavity for signs of dental abnormalities or disease and use appropriate techniques, as prescribed by the veterinarian, to promote and assist in maintaining dental health.**
- The student demonstrates knowledge of normal dentition, normal anatomy of the oral cavity, and normal occlusion.

- The student shows familiarity with a common system of tooth identification, such as the modified Triadan system.

- The student displays the ability to accurately identify common malocclusions, retained deciduous teeth, missing and supernumerary teeth, and evaluate other common oral pathologies, including periodontal disease, tooth fractures, and oral tumors.
- The student demonstrates understanding of proper dental terminology and abbreviations on dental charts and patients' medical records.
- The student displays an understanding of the importance of oral home care, the types of products available, and their proper applications.

71) **The student properly performs dental prophylaxis (manual and machine) in accordance with contemporary standards of care (Holstrom, et al., 2013).**

- The student wears proper safety equipment, including, but not limited to, mask or face shield, eye protection, gloves, dosimeter and protection from radiation.
- The student demonstrates understanding of the importance of general anesthesia with endotracheal intubation in the assessment and treatment of the canine and feline dental patient (AVDC, 2015). The student shows knowledge that according to the 2013 AAHA guidelines: "Cleaning a companion animal's teeth without general anesthesia is considered unacceptable and below the standard of care" (Holstrom, et al., 2013).
- The student displays an understanding of why dental radiography is essential to the accurate assessment of the patient's oral health.
- The student is aware of the patient's needs and status at all times while carefully monitoring anesthesia.
- The student makes certain the ET tube is correctly positioned and inflated and the nasopharynx is packed with absorbent gauze, so that the airway remains patent and the aspiration of water, blood, bacteria, and debris is prevented. The student deflates the cuff prior to repositioning or removing the ET tube and makes certain that pharyngeal packing material is removed when the procedure is completed.
- The student positions the animal properly, ensuring that the patient's head and neck are appropriately supported to prevent injury.
- The student uses towels and appropriate warming devices to prevent hypothermia.
- The student correctly identifies and appropriately uses hand instruments, holding them in a modified pen grasp.

- The student correctly uses the periodontal probe to measure the depth of the gingival sulcus or periodontal pocket.
- The student correctly uses the explorer to detect subgingival calculus, surface irregularities, or pulp exposure in fractured or worn (damaged) teeth.
- When using the ultrasonic scaler, the student uses the appropriate power setting and technique to scale both supragingivally and subgingivally for removal of plaque and calculus.
- The student properly positions and utilizes curettes on the tooth surface to remove supragingival plaque and to remove calculus from the root surface.
- The student correctly and appropriately uses dental machines, such as ultrasonic scalers. When using an ultrasonic scaler, the student correctly adjusts the water flow and power, is careful to use a light sweeping stroke across the tooth surface, using only the side of the tip, and limits contact to a maximum of 5–10 seconds per tooth to avoid thermal damage.
- After scaling, the student correctly uses the polisher, rubber polishing cup and appropriate "prophy paste" to thoroughly polish all surfaces both supragingivally and subgingivally to remove microscopic scratches. The student uses slow speeds (no more than 3,500 rpm), uses light pressure to flare the cup, and limits contact to a maximum of 5–10 seconds per tooth to avoid thermal damage.
- The student thoroughly rinses the teeth, gingival sulci, and/or periodontal pockets, carefully inspecting and cleaning any debris from the animal's mouth and face, while protecting the eyes at all times.
- The student makes certain to inform the veterinarian of any oral pathology that exists, including but not limited to fractured, discolored, missing, or mobile teeth, areas of excessive bleeding or inflammation and oral masses.
- The student correctly cleans, sharpens, disinfects, and sterilizes hand instruments.
- The student correctly cleans and maintains dental machines according to the manufacturer's recommendations.

72) **The student demonstrates knowledge of proper at-home care of the oral cavity.**

- The student demonstrates knowledge of how to educate clients about proper home care and displays the ability to explain it to them in an understandable manner that is likely to foster compliance.

- The student shows understanding of the need to use products specially formulated for animal use, with an emphasis on those with proven efficacy, rather than human products that may be harmful to animals and/or not designed to be swallowed.

- The student displays knowledge of the mechanisms by which home care products work and demonstrates the ability to make recommendations based on this information.

References

American Veterinary Dental College. (2015). *Information for Pet Owners*. Retrieved 2016, from www.avdc.org: www.avdc.org/dentalscaling.html (accessed September 14, 2016).

Fletcher, D., Boller, M., Brainard, B., Haskins, S., Hopper, K., McMichael, M., ... Smarick, S. (2012, June). RECOVER evidence and knowledge gap analysis on veterinary CPR. Part 7: Clinical guidelines. *J Vet Emerg Crit Care*, 22(Supplement 1), S103–S131.

Holstrom, S., Bellows, J., Juriga, S., Knutson, K., Niemiec, B., and Perrone, J. (2013). 2013 AAHA dental care guidelines for dogs and cats. *J Am Anim Hosp Assoc*, 75–92.

4

Anesthesia

Laurie J. Buell and Lisa E. Schenkel

4.1 Perioperative Management of the Veterinary Patient

1) **The student demonstrates the ability to work with the veterinarian to accurately evaluate the physical status and anesthetic risk of individual patients.**

- The student displays understanding that general anesthesia is an inherently compromised state that is produced by drugs that depress the CNS. As such, general anesthesia carries attendant risks of complications, primarily due to adverse physiologic changes to the nervous system, cardiovascular system, and central nervous system function.
- The student shows knowledge of the American Society of Anesthesiologists (ASA) classification of patient physical status (Brodbelt, Flaherty, and Pettifer, 2015).
- The student demonstrates understanding that the patient's potential for survival of general anesthesia is, in part, determined by the individual animal's physical status.
- The student shows awareness that the animal's physical status is determined by signalment, patient history, physical examination, diagnostic tests, and the procedure to be performed.
- The student demonstrates understanding that the animal's anesthetic risk often is affected by signalment (species, breed, age, weight, reproductive status, temperament, etc.). For example, brachycephalic breeds often have partially obstructed airways due to structural abnormalities. Neonatal animals are prone to hypothermia, dehydration and hypoglycemia, as well as a decreased ability to biotransform drugs due to immature liver function. Geriatric animals may be less able to biotransform and excrete drugs due to decreased liver and/or kidney function. The student shows knowledge that the animal's weight must be accurate because it determines drug dosages, fluid administration rates and, often, the type of anesthetic system used (rebreathing vs non-rebreathing).

- The student appropriately works with the veterinarian to gather as much information as possible on the patient relevant to anesthesia prior to and during the pre-anesthetic period.

2) **Based on the individual patient's physical status, anesthetic risk and type of procedure, the student demonstrates the ability to work with the veterinarian to tailor anesthetic and analgesic regimens to meet the needs of individual patients, with the goals of maximizing safety, while minimizing and/or preventing nociception and pain.**

- The student accurately defines the terms "anesthesia, general anesthesia, surgical anesthesia, balanced (multimodal) anesthesia, local anesthesia, regional anesthesia, and dissociative anesthesia." The student demonstrates understanding of the appropriate clinical applications of each.
- The student displays understanding of the pre-anesthetic period as time to anticipate potential complications, attempt to optimize the animal's condition and take proactive steps to prevent complications from arising. For example, the student demonstrates awareness that brachycephalic breeds generally need very rapid anesthetic induction, intubation and anesthetic recovery (to maintain patent airways), and very close monitoring following extubation. As another example, the student takes special care to closely monitor the body temperature of neonates and keep them warm, preparing appropriate warming devices, such as hot water circulating blankets, Bair huggers® and/or Hot Dog® patient warming systems. Even in emergency procedures, the student displays awareness that, if time allows, all steps should be taken to correct and stabilize the following conditions prior to anesthetic induction: dehydration, hypovolemia, hypotension, anemia, hypoproteinemia, cardiac dysfunction, respiratory distress, renal dysfunction, clotting defects, and hyperthermia or hypothermia.

Assessing Essential Skills of Veterinary Technology Students, Third Edition. Edited by Laurie J. Buell, Lisa E. Schenkel and Sabrina Timperman.
© 2017 John Wiley & Sons, Inc. Published 2017 by John Wiley & Sons, Inc.
Companion website: www.wiley.com/go/buell/skills

- Following the veterinarian's orders, the student secures venous access during the pre-anesthetic period to provide an administration route for emergency drugs, if needed, as well as to administer fluids to prevent and/or treat dehydration and/or hypotension and to speed the rate of drug elimination.
- Following the veterinarian's orders, the student fasts patients and withholds water for the appropriate time periods prior to anesthetic induction. The student displays awareness that birds, neonates and exotic animals may be fasted for very short periods or not at all due to their tendency to become hypoglycemic. The student also displays awareness that fasting species that are hind-gut fermenters, such as rabbits and guinea pigs, can lead to gastrointestinal ileus.
- The student displays awareness that only the veterinarian may prescribe anesthetic agents, doses and routes of administration. However, the student shows understanding that it is the technician's/technologist's duty to make appropriate suggestions and communicate pertinent observations to the supervising veterinarian.
- The student displays awareness that no pre-anesthetic, anesthetic or analgesic agent is free from adverse effects and that no single agent is safe for all animals. The student, therefore, demonstrates understanding that determination of pre-anesthetic, anesthetic and analgesic protocols should be tailored to the individual patient based on: patient's signalment, physical status, co-morbidities, type and duration of procedure, existing and anticipated pain level, inpatient versus outpatient, elective versus emergency procedures, and the veterinarian's and technician's/technologist's experience.

3) **The student accurately calculates dosages of agents administered during the peri-anesthetic period.**
   - During the pre-anesthetic period (on the day of the procedure), the student accurately weighs the patient and records the weight in the patient's record.
   - The student correctly calculates doses of anesthetic and analgesic drugs based on the patient's weight, when appropriate.
     a) The student shows awareness that, in overweight animals, doses of anesthetic-related drugs should be calculated based on lean body weight, rather than actual body weight.
     b) The student displays awareness that doses of anesthetic-related drugs should be reduced in emaciated animals.

- The student correctly prepares and accurately measures doses of enterally and parenterally administered anesthetic and analgesic agents.
- The student correctly documents calculated doses in patient records.
  a) The student accurately records the calculated doses of drugs in correct units of measure, for example, in grams (g), milligrams (mg), micrograms (mcg), International Units (IU), or milliequivalents (mEq).
  b) The student displays awareness that the dosage strength of the drug (e.g., mg/ml, mg/tab) must be included when recording the dosage form of the drug (e.g., number of oral tablets or number of ml of an injectable solution).
  c) For agents administered "to effect," the student uses "drawn/given" method, writing on the patient's record both the amount of drug drawn up and the amount actually administered. For controlled drugs, the student uses the "drawn/given" method in the controlled substances log.

4) **The student demonstrates the ability to properly administer pre-anesthetic, anesthetic and analgesic agents by appropriate routes, including anesthetic induction by injectable agents, as well as the administration of anesthetic gases and oxygen by mask and endotracheal tube.**
   - The student demonstrates basic understanding of appropriate uses, major contraindications, common adverse effects, and appropriate routes and methods of administration for commonly used, injectable anesthetic and pre-anesthetic agents, and their reversal agents, where applicable.
   - The student demonstrates basic understanding of properties, appropriate uses, major contraindications and common adverse effects of inhalant anesthetic agents, such as isoflurane and sevoflurane.
   - The student demonstrates understanding of relative advantages and disadvantages of the various methods of anesthetic induction, and utilizes each appropriately. The student displays awareness that mask inductions permit anesthetic induction without IV access and may be warranted in individual cases. However, the student displays knowledge of disadvantages associated with mask inductions, including but not limited to: lack of airway control, increased dead space, prolonged Stage II (compared with intravenously administered induction agents), increased patient stress and increased atmospheric pollution with anesthetic gas.
   - The student demonstrates the ability to properly administer injectable anesthetic-related drugs by bolus and/or constant rate infusion.

- The student demonstrates the ability to administer inhalant anesthetic agents by mask and endotracheal tube.
- The student correctly records the dose as well as the time and route of administration of anesthetic-related agents used in the anesthetic record.

5) **The student demonstrates the ability to endotracheally intubate patients correctly and safely.**

- The student demonstrates knowledge of the advantages of endotracheal intubation, such as reducing dead space, decreasing exposure of personnel to waste gases, maintaining a patent airway, allowing assisted or controlled ventilation, and decreasing risk of aspiration of vomitus, saliva, and/or blood (when the cuff is inflated).
- The student displays understanding of the potential complications of overly aggressive intubation or overinflation of the cuff, including but not limited to, endotracheal inflammation, necrosis or tracheal rupture; trauma to the soft palate, pharynx or larynx; stimulation of the vagus nerve, potentially leading to bradycardia or other cardiac dysrhythmias; and/or damage to the recurrent laryngeal nerve, potentially leading to laryngeal paralysis and/or bradycardia. The student shows awareness of the need to avoid laryngeal trauma, particularly in cats, to avoid laryngospasm.
- The student demonstrates awareness that underinflation of the cuff dilutes the percentage of inhalant anesthetic reaching the gas exchange portion of the lungs, as well as increasing the risk of aspiration.
- The student selects the appropriate size and diameter endotracheal (ET) tube. The student demonstrates awareness that the distal end of tube should not extend beyond the level of thoracic inlet.
  a) The student pre-measures the distance from incisors to the cervical trachea near the thoracic inlet.
  b) To minimize mechanical dead space, the student avoids use of an overly long ET tube, making certain the connector is very near the incisors.
  c) The student demonstrates understanding that too narrow a diameter or too long an ET tube increases resistance to breathing.
- The student accurately identifies the anesthetic depth (stage and plane of anesthesia) at which intubation is appropriate. For example, the student shows awareness that laryngospasm may result when intubation is attempted in a cat at too light an anesthetic plane.
- In placing the ET tube, the student carefully avoids overly aggressive intubation, underinflation and overinflation of the cuff.

- The student checks to insure proper placement of the ET tube by ausculting the lungs and ensuring that breath sounds are present in all lung fields. The student shows awareness that proper ET tube placement also can be confirmed by capnography.
- The student secures the ET tube in place in a manner suitable for the species and type of procedure.
- The student regularly monitors for proper cuff inflation, obstruction or movement of the ET tube. The student deflates the cuff prior to repositioning or removing the ET tube.
- The student safely extubates the patient at the appropriate time (generally when oral and pharyngeal reflexes have returned) to avoid chewing on the tube by the patient.

6) **Based on observation of clinical signs and the correct use of monitoring equipment, the student demonstrates the ability to accurately monitor the patient's status throughout all stages of the procedure.**

- The student demonstrates understanding of the essential components of anesthesia, including, but not limited to, the pre-anesthetic period, anesthetic induction, maintenance and recovery; anesthetic monitoring; and pain assessment and pain management.
- The student shows awareness of the patient's ongoing status before, during and after anesthesia to provide for adequate anesthesia, analgesia and safe recovery. The student does not leave the animal unobserved during the peri-anesthetic and anesthetic periods, including following administration of pre-anesthetic medications as well as anesthetic recovery after extubation.
- The student shows understanding that the physiologic status of the anesthetized patient is evaluated through assessment of respiratory, cardiovascular, and central nervous system function.
  a) The student demonstrates knowledge of values for vital signs, neuromuscular signs (degree of muscle tone) and CNS reflexes (e.g., swallowing, palpebral, pedal, corneal) associated with each phase of CNS depression (and/or each stage of anesthesia).
  b) The student shows familiarity with acceptable values for vital signs, neuromuscular signs, and CNS reflexes in awake and recovering animals.
- The student demonstrates understanding that, for ASA Status I or II patients, a veterinarian or veterinary technician/technologist should be continuously present with and focused on assessing the patient's respiratory, cardiovascular, and CNS function. The student shows awareness that, if this is not possible, patient status should be monitored a

minimum of every 5 minutes during anesthesia and throughout the recovery period (American College of Veterinary Anesthesiologists, 2009).

- The student shows understanding that, for ASA Status III, IV, or V patients, or for any horse anesthetized with an inhalant anesthetic, or for any horse anesthetized for longer than 45 minutes, a veterinarian or veterinary technician/technologist should be continuously present with the patient and focused on assessing the patient's respiratory, cardiovascular, and CNS function, during anesthesia and throughout the recovery period (American College of Veterinary Anesthesiologists, 2009).

- The student demonstrates understanding of the importance of maintaining an anesthetic record for each patient, both as legal documentation of significant events and to facilitate identification of trends in monitored values, thereby allowing early recognition of potential complications.

- The student accurately records parameters in the anesthetic record a minimum of every 5 minutes.

- The student displays awareness that monitoring equipment is not a reliable replacement for the technician's eyes, ears, and hands. As much as is practical, the student uses their senses to monitor vital signs, muscle tone, and reflexes, including, but not limited to: direct palpation of pulse rate and strength; auscultation of the chest with a stethoscope for heart rate and rhythm and the presence of abnormal respiratory sounds; observation of the animal's chest and reservoir bag for respiratory rate and depth; monitoring capillary refill time, mucous membrane color, and body temperature; and checking muscle tone and reflexes to help assess the level of CNS depression. The student displays knowledge of acceptable values for all parameters, both awake and under anesthesia.

- The student uses appropriate monitoring equipment to aid in assessing patient status at all times during and following the procedure. The student displays the ability to: use a stethoscope and differentiate normal from abnormal heart sounds; use a blood pressure monitor and differentiate acceptable arterial blood pressures from hypo- or hypertension; and use an electrocardiograph and differentiate normal from abnormal ECGs. The student demonstrates the ability to use a pulse oximeter and a capnometer/capnograph to assess the adequacy of oxygenation and ventilation.

7) **The student demonstrates understanding of how to assess the patient for evidence of nociception and/or pain, administer analgesic therapy properly and in accordance with the veterinarian's orders, and carefully monitor the efficacy of analgesic therapy.**

- The student demonstrates familiarity with the difference between physiologic and pathologic pain.

- The student correctly defines terms such as "visceral pain, deep somatic pain, superficial somatic pain, adaptive pain, maladaptive pain, neuropathic pain, and inflammatory pain."

- The student demonstrates knowledge of the physiological process of nociception and pain perception.

   a) The student correctly explains the physiological events leading to central and peripheral sensitization.

   b) The student accurately describes the terms "hyperalgesia" and "allodynia."

   c) The student explains the clinical implications of maladaptive pain in developing effective pain management protocols.

- The student displays knowledge of physiological signs of pain resulting from reflex ventilatory, cardiovascular, and hormonal responses to nociception. The student demonstrates awareness that objective signs of pain, including increases in respiratory rate, heart rate, arterial blood pressure, catecholamine, and cortisol levels, are not necessarily correlated with the intensity of pain sensation (Buell, 1999; Cambridge, Tobias, and Newberry, 2000; Holton, Scott, Nolan, Reid, and Welsh, 1998; Fox and Mellor, 1998).

- The student demonstrates knowledge of obvious behaviors associated with pain, such as vocalization, resentment of palpation, trembling, reluctance to move or bear weight, self-mutilation, hunched-up posture, and so on. However, the student demonstrates awareness that vocalization is not necessarily correlated with pain intensity, lack of obvious pain behaviors does not indicate lack of pain, and behavioral signs of pain may be very subtle, making very close monitoring essential (Hansen and Hardie, 1993; Hardie, Hansen, and Carroll, 1997; Hellyer and Gaynor, 1998).

- The student demonstrates knowledge of normal behaviors characteristic of particular species and breeds. The student also shows awareness of behaviors induced by pain in particular species and breeds. For example, lack of grooming or over-grooming a specific area may be an indication of pain in cats, while kicking at the abdomen may be sign of pain in horses.

- The student shows awareness that deviation from the individual animal's normal behaviors may be evidence of pain (e.g., inability to sleep, anorexia, depression, apprehensiveness, or a normally friendly animal behaving aggressively or unwilling to interact) (Hansen and Hardie, 1993; Hardie,

Hansen, and Carroll, 1997; Hellyer and Gaynor, 1998).

- The student demonstrates knowledge of how the effects of drugs, such as tranquilizers and anesthetic agents, can interfere with accurate pain assessment. For example, an animal who has been sedated may not exhibit pain-induced behaviors but still be experiencing significant pain.
- The student displays knowledge of potentially detrimental physiological effects of pain, including diminished wound healing, impaired immune system function, and the release of proinflammatory cytokines (Wiese, Muir, and Wittum, 2005; Quandt, Lee, and Powell, 2005).
- The student demonstrates awareness that the effects of not treating pain often are more deleterious than the potential adverse effects associated with recommended dosages of analgesic drugs (Wiese, Muir, and Wittum, 2005).
- The student displays awareness that, as an adjunct to thorough patient evaluation, appropriate use of pain scales is necessary in ensuring that pain is properly assessed and treated.
- The student demonstrates understanding of how to judge the efficacy of pain therapy in the individual animal, based on reduction of behaviors associated with pain, as well as return to more normal behavior for the individual animal.
- The student shows understanding of the concepts of analgesia, pre-emptive analgesia and balanced analgesia.
- The student demonstrates basic understanding of the appropriate uses, major contraindications, common adverse effects, and appropriate routes and methods of administration for commonly-used analgesic agents. These may include, but are not limited to, opioid analgesic agents (and their reversal agents), non-steroidal anti-inflammatory agents, NMDA-receptor antagonists (such as ketamine), alpha$_2$ agonists (and their reversal agents), and local anesthetic agents.
- The student displays knowledge of how to implement appropriate pain management protocols, while continuing to monitor the patient's ongoing status. The student demonstrates knowledge that any animal given analgesic agents must be closely monitored for adverse effects in the pre-anesthetic period, the anesthetic period, and the entire recovery period.

8) **The student demonstrates the ability to detect anesthetic complications and respond to them quickly and appropriately.**
   - The student shows awareness of the importance of being proactive in managing the anesthetized patient by anticipating likely complications and taking appropriate steps to avoid them.
   - The student demonstrates knowledge of how to take steps to avoid and closely monitor for the presence of abnormalities, potential complications, and/or clinically significant changes in patient status that may arise during the anesthetic and/or peri-anesthetic period.
   - The student displays awareness of the need to immediately inform the supervisor/veterinarian of any anesthetic complications.
   - The student demonstrates knowledge of how to address complications rapidly and appropriately.
   - The student displays understanding of how to rapidly recognize and respond to respiratory complications. For example, the student shows awareness of an SpO_2 of <95% as evidence of hypoxemia. The student displays knowledge of common causes of hypoxemia during anesthesia, including, but not limited to, inadequate O_2 flow, loss of airway or obstruction of the breathing circuit. The student demonstrates knowledge of malfunctions in oxygen supply, anesthetic machine, ET tube and/or breathing circuit that may lead to inadequate oxygenation and/or ventilation. The student shows knowledge of how to rapidly check each potential cause and take immediate corrective action. In addition, the student displays awareness of how to anticipate adverse respiratory effects commonly associated with various anesthetic-related and analgesic agents, quickly recognize them, and respond appropriately. For example, the student shows awareness that propofol administration is associated with risk of apnea, particularly with too rapid administration. If this were to occur, the student demonstrates knowledge of how to administer positive pressure ventilations with oxygen until the animal resumes spontaneous respiration. In addition, the student displays knowledge of how to recognize hypoventilation and take appropriate remedial steps, such as reducing the vaporizer setting to the minimum anesthetic depth needed to perform the procedure, correctly administering positive-pressure ventilations (assisting or controlling ventilation), and addressing the cause of hypoventilation, when possible, while alerting the veterinarian.
   - The student demonstrates knowledge of how to rapidly recognize and respond to cardiovascular complications, such as cardiac dysrhythmias. The student shows appreciation of the importance of being proactive by anticipating adverse cardiovascular effects commonly associated with various anesthetic-related and analgesic agents; quickly recognizing them; and responding appropriately.

For example, if an alpha$_2$-adrenoreceptor agonist is administered, the student shows awareness of bradycardia as a common adverse effect and demonstrates awareness of the need to have the correct reversal agent prepared and ready to administer on the veterinarian's order.

- The student displays awareness of hypotension as a common anesthetic complication and shows understanding of how to recognize clinically significant blood pressure abnormalities. The student demonstrates knowledge of compensatory responses which may occur in response to hypotension, including increased heart rate and vasomotor tone, leading to abnormalities in mucous membrane color, capillary refill time, urine output, and/or body temperature. The student demonstrates awareness of the need to have appropriate IV fluids (and/or blood products) and pressor and/or positive inotropic agents prepared and ready to administer on the veterinarian's order. The student shows understanding of how to carefully monitor fluid administration rates and shows familiarity with signs of overhydration.

- The student shows awareness of the need to closely monitor body temperature during the peri-anesthetic period. The student displays knowledge of common causes of hypothermia and how to take appropriate preventative steps, particularly in neonate and pediatric patients. If hypothermia does occur, the student shows knowledge of how to recognize it and take appropriate therapeutic measures, including use of IV fluids warmed to body temperature, Bair huggers®, Hot Dog® warming systems, circulating warm water blankets, and so on. The student shows awareness of common causes of hyperthermia during the peri-anesthetic period (including malignant hyperthermia) and displays knowledge of how to take appropriate therapeutic measures, including use of fans, tepid water baths and enemas, and so on.

- The student demonstrates knowledge of how to promptly recognize neuromuscular indicators of excessive CNS depression, for example, profound muscle relaxation, weak pupillary light reflexes, and centered, dilated pupils.

9) **The student demonstrates knowledge of how to respond appropriately to anesthetic emergencies, including correctly administering reversal agents and emergency drugs, as ordered by the veterinarian, and effectively performing suitable resuscitation procedures.**

- The student shows awareness of how to promptly recognize potentially life-threatening anesthetic complications, including signs of respiratory arrest and cardiopulmonary arrest. The student demonstrates recognition of the need to immediately inform the supervisor/veterinarian.

- The student demonstrates appreciation of the need to make certain that anesthetic reversal agents, emergency drugs and equipment, and crash cart are prepared and readily available in advance of the procedure.

- The student displays the ability to accurately calculate doses and administer appropriate emergency drugs and/or anesthetic reversal agents (i.e., specific antagonists).

- The student demonstrates awareness that emergency drug doses for each patient should be calculated prior to anesthetic induction.

- The student shows knowledge of how to secure a patent airway and correctly administer positive-pressure ventilations with oxygen by anesthetic machine or resuscitation bag (Ambu® bag). The student demonstrates knowledge of how to properly perform CPR, according to current standards.

- The student demonstrates the ability to properly complete a controlled substance log according to applicable federal and state regulations.

4.2 Management and Use of Anesthetic Equipment

10) **The student properly operates and cares for anesthetic equipment and monitoring instruments, demonstrating the ability to detect and appropriately address equipment malfunction or failure.**

- Given the requirements of the anesthetic protocol and individual patient, the student selects the appropriate anesthetic machine, breathing circuit, and monitoring instruments.

- In advance of the procedure, the student completes a pre-anesthetic check list of all anesthetic delivery and monitoring instruments to make certain that all equipment is in proper working order and free of leaks.

- The student demonstrates the ability to correctly operate and adjust the anesthetic machine and monitoring equipment.

- The student is alert to and responds appropriately to equipment malfunctions or improper equipment set-up.

11) **The student demonstrates understanding of the clinical significance of pulse oximetry and correctly operates and cares for pulse oximeters.**

- The student correctly sets up and operates the pulse oximeter, properly placing the probe.

- The student shows understanding that accurate pulse oximeter readings are dependent on placing the probe on a well-perfused area.
- The student demonstrates understanding that pulse oximetry may be used to assess adequacy of oxygenation because pulse oximetry measures arterial hemoglobin saturation with oxygen as SpO_2 or SaO_2.
- The student shows knowledge of acceptable SpO_2 or SaO_2 levels, and correctly differentiates them from hypoxemia.
- The student displays awareness of the causes of inaccurate readings, such as vasoconstriction, motion, pressure of the clip interfering with capillary blood flow, hypotension, or severe bradycardia (when the heart rate is too low to distinguish between arterial and venous blood flow).
- The student properly cares for the pulse oximeter, following the manufacturer's recommendations for cleaning and maintenance, keeping it ready for use when needed.

12) **The student shows appreciation of the clinical significance of capnometry and capnography and correctly operates and cares for the capnometer and capnograph.**
    - The student correctly differentiates between a capnometer and a capnograph, showing understanding that a capnometer measures the amount of CO_2 in inspired and expired air, while the capnograph produces the graphical record of the CO_2 concentration.
    - The student demonstrates understanding that assessing the adequacy of ventilation requires measurement of CO_2 levels either in the blood or expired air. Therefore, capnometry can be used to evaluate the adequacy of ventilation.
    - The student shows understanding of end-tidal CO_2 ($ETCO_2$) as measurement of CO_2 in expired air at the end of expiration. The student demonstrates knowledge of acceptable $ETCO_2$ levels in anesthetized animals.
    - The student displays the ability to use the capnometer/capnograph correctly and differentiate acceptable $ETCO_2$ levels from hypo- and hypercapnia. The student demonstrates awareness that high $ETCO_2$ levels may indicate hypoventilation, a common anesthetic complication in spontaneously breathing patients. The student demonstrates awareness that low $ETCO_2$ levels indicate hyperventilation, most often seen with overzealous artificial or mechanical ventilation (Thomas and Lerche, 2011).
    - The student displays knowledge that hypoventilation may lead to respiratory acidosis, while hyperventilation may lead to respiratory alkalosis.
    - The student shows fundamental understanding of the physiologic basis of the components of the capnographic waveform. For example, in the normal waveform, the baseline represents inspiration because atmospheric air normally contains insignificant amounts of CO_2.
    - The student shows awareness of common technical errors that lead to decreased $ETCO_2$ levels, such as endotracheal tube or breathing circuit obstruction, or disconnection of the endotracheal tube from the breathing circuit. The student shows awareness of common technical errors that lead to increased $ETCO_2$ levels, including depleted CO_2 absorber (Thomas and Lerche, 2011).
    - The student displays understanding of the difference between mainstream and sidestream capnometers and the potential advantages and disadvantages of each.
    - The student correctly cares for capnometers/ capnographs, following the manufacturer's recommendations for maintenance and calibration, and keeping them ready for use when needed.

13) **The student properly places, utilizes, and cares for the esophageal stethoscope.**
    - After the patient is intubated, the student properly lubricates the tube of and inserts the esophageal stethoscope, advancing it until an audible heartbeat is detected.
    - The student correctly uses the esophageal stethoscope to aid in assessing heart rate and rhythm. The student demonstrates the ability to recognize the presence of abnormal heart sounds.
    - The student displays awareness of the potential for the esophageal stethoscope to act as a fomite. The student properly cleans and cares for the esophageal stethoscope, following the manufacturer's recommendations, and keeping it ready for use when needed.

14) **The student correctly performs electrocardiography and properly cares for the electrocardiograph.**
    - The student correctly sets up and operates the electrocardiograph, properly placing leads and applying electrode gel or alcohol, as needed.
    - The student demonstrates ability to recognize normal sinus rhythm (NSR) and to differentiate NSR from cardiac dysrhythmias.
    - The student displays the ability to recognize cardiac dysrhythmias commonly associated with the peri-anesthetic period, for example, sinus bradycardia, sinus tachycardia, atrioventricular block, and ventricular premature contractions.
    - The student shows understanding that the ECG monitors electrical activity of the heart only and does not indicate the pumping ability of the heart.

- The student displays the ability to distinguish abnormal tracings due to mechanical causes from those resulting from abnormal cardiac electrical activity. For example, the student shows familiarity with ECG tracings due to 60-cycle interference.
- The student demonstrates the ability to appropriately and promptly respond to cardiac dysrhythmias that occur during the peri-anesthetic period. For example, if an anesthetized animal were to exhibit sinus tachycardia, the student shows knowledge of the potential causes, including but not limited to, nociception, hypotension, hypercapnia, hypoxia or possibly even inadequate anesthetic depth. The student shows awareness that the appropriate response is to evaluate and address each potential cause.
- The student properly maintains the electrocardiograph, following the manufacturer's recommendations, keeping it prepared for use when needed.

15) **The student demonstrates knowledge of, correctly operates and cares for anesthetic machines, breathing circuits, and face masks.**
    - The student demonstrates knowledge of the properties, appropriate uses, major contraindications, and common adverse effects of inhalant anesthetic agents.
    - The student demonstrates functional knowledge of and properly operates all components of the anesthetic machine and anesthetic breathing systems, including, but not limited to, the flowmeter, vaporizer, rebreathing bags, adjustable pressure-limiting valve (pop-off valve), carbon dioxide absorber canister, oxygen flush valve, pressure manometer, flutter valves, hoses, Y piece, scavenging systems, and activated charcoal canisters (for waste anesthetic gases).
    - The student makes certain that the reservoir bag is about 75% full at peak expiration. The student displays knowledge of reasons why a reservoir bag would not remain properly inflated (e.g., too low an oxygen flow rate). The student shows understanding of why a reservoir bag would become overinflated (e.g., if it is too small for the patient or if the pop-off valve is closed).
    - The student regularly cleans and disinfects all parts of the anesthetic machine, including flutter valves, according to the manufacturer's recommendations. After each use, the student thoroughly washes, rinses, and air dries breathing circuits, including reservoir bags.
    - The student performs daily safety inspection of all anesthetic equipment, including, but not limited to, checking pressure gauges to make certain gas cylinders contain adequate gas, checking the

anesthetic machine and breathing circuits for leaks, checking the CO_2 absorber is fresh and the vaporizer is full. The student rechecks all equipment after each procedure.
- The student uses an appropriate breathing system for each individual animal (i.e., non-rebreathing systems are not recommended for animals weighing more than 10 kg) (Mosley, 2015). The student demonstrates understanding of advantages and disadvantages of each type of breathing system. The student sets an oxygen flow rate appropriate for the individual animal and for the breathing system.
- The student uses an appropriate size rebreathing bag for the individual patient (i.e., a minimum of 60 ml/kg or six times the patient's tidal volume) (Thomas and Lerche, 2011).
- The student correctly uses face masks. The student demonstrates understanding of disadvantages associated with induction by face mask, including increased contamination of room air with anesthetic gases. To minimize environmental contamination with anesthetic gases, the student shows knowledge of measures such as using well-fitting face masks only in well ventilated areas.

16) **The student demonstrates knowledge of and correctly cares for endotracheal tubes.**
    - The student displays knowledge of different types of endotracheal tubes (e.g., Murphy, Cole, etc.), their construction (e.g., rubber, polyvinyl chloride, silicone) and parts (e.g., connector, cuff, valve, radiopaque marker, bevel, valve, etc.), how they are sized (internal diameter), and appropriate uses of each type.
    - The student thoroughly cleans the inside and outside of the ET tube with mild detergent solution after each use, with the cuff sufficiently inflated to remove all debris within the folds. The student very thoroughly rinses the tube in warm water until no detergent residue remains. The student sufficiently air dries the tube, with the cuff inflated, to promote desiccation of microorganisms.
    - The student shows awareness that residues of many disinfectants, such as chlorhexidine, glutaraldehyde and ethylene oxide, remaining in ET tubes are associated with tracheal mucosal injury (Veterinary Anesthesia and Analgesia Support Group, 2016; McKelvey and Hollingshead, 2003).
    - After each use, the student inspects the tube for patency and signs of damage. The student inflates the cuff to make certain inflation is symmetrical and sustained. The student makes certain to discard any damaged ET tubes and ensures that adequate numbers of replacements are available.

17) **The student correctly uses anesthetic machines and resuscitation bags (e.g., Ambu® bags) to administer positive-pressure ventilations to the patient.**
   - The student properly connects resuscitation bags to oxygen sources to deliver 100% oxygen to the patient. When an oxygen source is unavailable, the student correctly uses a resuscitation bag to deliver room air.
   - The student uses an appropriate size resuscitation bag for the patient.
   - When using an Ambu® bag, the student ensures that the patient's chest rises to the same extent as with a normal, awake inspiration.
   - When administering positive-pressure ventilations with an anesthetic machine, the student correctly monitors inspiratory pressure, using the pressure manometer. The student makes certain that peak inspiratory pressure does not exceed $20\,cm\,H_2O$ in healthy small animals (Muir, Hubbell, Bednarski, and Lerche, 2013). The student displays awareness of adverse effects of exceeding maximal inspiratory pressure and takes care not to overinflate lungs.
   - The student makes certain that the pop-off valve is closed during inspiration and open during expiration.
   - The student applies pressure to and releases the bag such that the inspiratory to expiratory ratio is 1:2. For example, if inspiration is 1 second, then the animal is given 2 seconds to exhale. The student ensures that the manometer reads "0" during expiration.
   - The student correctly uses a pulse oximeter and a capnometer/capnograph to guide the rate of positive pressure ventilations.

18) **The student demonstrates knowledge of, correctly operates and maintains waste gas scavenging systems.**
   - The student demonstrates awareness of active systems (in which a fan or vacuum pump draws waste gas into the scavenger) and passive scavenging systems (in which gas pressure in the anesthetic machine drives the gas into the scavenger). The student shows understanding that the waste gas must be vented to the outdoors in a way that prevents waste gases from reentering any part of the facility.
   - The student makes certain that the waste gas scavenging system is properly connected to the adjustable pressure-limiting valve (pop-off valve).
   - In a facility with an active system, the student makes certain the system is turned on daily and the scavenger is prevented from excessively drawing gases from the breathing circuit (causing collapse of the rebreathing bag).
   - The student makes certain that the waste gas scavenging system is working properly and is not blocked.
   - In facilities using activated charcoal canisters (such as F/AIR™ anesthesia gas filters), the student replaces the canister after a maximum of 12–15 hours of use or when the weight of canister has increased by 50 g over its initial weight.
   - The student is aware that activated charcoal canisters do not absorb nitrous oxide and are relatively inefficient at oxygen flow rates higher than 2 L/min (McKelvey and Hollingshead, 2003; Thomas and Lerche, 2011).

19) **The student demonstrates knowledge of, correctly uses and cares for sources of oxygen and other gases.**
   - The student demonstrates functional knowledge of oxygen and other gas sources, including gas cylinders, oxygen concentrators and gas lines. For common oxygen tank sizes, including E, H, and T tanks, the student demonstrates knowledge of the relationship between pressure and content. The student displays understanding of the functions of pressure gauges and reads them correctly.
   - The student displays knowledge of the functions of and correct settings for pressure regulators (pressure-reducing valves).
   - The student properly identifies gas cylinders, gas lines, and outlets by color coding. The student demonstrates understanding of the cylinder yoke and pin-indexed safety system.
   - The student correctly attaches gas cylinders and gas lines to the anesthetic machine.
   - The student regularly checks pressure gauges to ensure adequate gas remains in tanks. The student is alert to abnormal readings on pressure gauges and responds appropriately.
   - The student demonstrates knowledge of the functions of O_2 flowmeters and operates them correctly.
   - The student properly stores gas cylinders so that they are attached to yokes, secured to specifically designed carts or chained to a wall, making certain they are kept in cool, dry areas. The student regularly checks cylinders and gas lines for defects.

20) **The student correctly operates and cares for blood pressure monitors.**
   - The student accurately defines the terms "systolic pressure, diastolic pressure, and mean arterial pressure." The student displays understanding of the clinical significance of those terms.

- The student shows awareness that direct monitors provide more accurate measurement of blood pressure than indirect monitors.
- The student displays knowledge of indirect blood pressure monitors, including oscillometric and Doppler devices. The student shows basic understanding of how these monitors measure blood pressure. The student shows awareness of inaccuracies associated with each type of monitor in smaller patients.
- The student correctly uses blood pressure monitoring devices to attain reasonably accurate measures of arterial blood pressure. The student selects a cuff of appropriate width (30–40% limb circumference), properly placing the cuff around an appendage or the tail. For the Doppler method, the student properly clips fur over the artery, places gel on the probe and places the probe over the artery, distal to the cuff.
- The student demonstrates knowledge of acceptable values for arterial blood pressure.
- The student correctly cares for and cleans blood pressure monitoring devices, following the manufacturer's recommendations.

21) **The student correctly uses and cares for laryngoscopes.**
- The student properly uses the laryngoscope, choosing a suitable blade for the size and species of animal and correctly positioning the blade.
- The student shows awareness that use of a laryngoscope is recommended for all intubations, even when intubation can be accomplished without it, because laryngoscope use allows oropharyngeal examination and reduces the risk of traumatic intubation (Mosley, 2015).
- The student makes certain the laryngoscope blade has been cleaned and disinfected/sterilized prior to use, according to the manufacturer's recommendations.
- The student properly cares for and maintains the laryngoscope and blades according to the manufacturer's recommendations. The student makes certain the laryngoscope is kept ready for use when needed, with batteries charged and the lamp or fiber optic light pipe replaced as needed.

22) **The student correctly uses and cares for temperature monitoring devices (e.g., thermometer, etc.).**
- The student correctly uses a variety of temperature monitoring devices, such as digital or liquid capillary (mercury or alcohol) thermometers and esophageal or rectal temperature probes.
- The student uses protective thermometer covers when taking a rectal temperature to reduce the risk of disease transmission (Rondeau and Hanie, 2014).
- When taking rectal temperature, the student applies appropriate lubricant and gently inserts the thermometer into the rectum in a manner that avoids tissue trauma.
- The student makes certain that temperature monitoring devices are appropriately cleaned/disinfected after each use.

References

American College of Veterinary Anesthesiologists (2009). *ACVA Monitoring Guidelines Update* Retrieved from the American College of Veterinary Anesthesia and Analgesia Web Site: www.acvaa.org (accessed September 14, 2016).

Brodbelt, D. C., Flaherty, D., and Pettifer, G. R. (2015). Anesthetic risk and informed consent. In: K. A. Grimm, L. A. Lamont, W. J. Tranquilli, S. A. Greene, and S. A. Robertson (Eds.), *Veterinary Anesthesia and Analgesia: The Fifth Edition of Lumb and Jones* (pp. 11–22). Ames: John Wiley & Sons, Inc.

Buell, L. J. (1999). *Postoperative Opioid Analgesia in Dogs and Cats: An Analysis of the Pharmacological and Clinical Effects of Strong Agonists Relative to Mixed Agonist-Antagonists [Master's Thesis].* Valhalla: New York Medical College.

Cambridge, A., Tobias, K., and Newberry, R. (2000). Subjective and objective measurement of postoperative pain in cats. *J Am Vet Med Assoc*, 217(5), 685–690.

Fox, S., and Mellor, D. L. (1998). Changes in plasma cortisol concentrations in bitches in response to different combinations of halothane and butorphanol, with or without ovariohysterectomy. *Res Vet Sci*, 125–133.

Grimm, K., Lamont, L., Tranquilli, W., Greene, S., and Robertson, S. (2015). *Veterinary Anesthesia and Analgesia: The Fifth Edition of Lumb and Jones.* Baltimore: John Wiley & Sons, Inc.

Hansen, B., and Hardie, E. (1993). Prescription and use of analgesics in dogs and cats in a veterinary teaching hospital: 258 cases. *J Am Vet Med Assoc*, 202(9), 1485–1494.

Hardie, E. M., Hansen, B. D., and Carroll, G. S. (1997). Behavior after ovariohysterectomy in the dog: what's normal? *Appl Anim Behav Sci*, 51, 111–128.

Hellyer, P. W., and Gaynor, J. S. (1998). Acute postsurgical pain in dogs and cats. *Compen Contin Educ Prac Vet*, 20(2), 140–153.

Holton, L. L., Scott, E. M., Nolan, A. M., Reid, J., and Welsh, E. (1998). Relationship between physiological factors and clinical pain in dogs scored using a numerical rating scale. *J Small Anim Pract*, 39(10), 469–474.

McKelvey, D., and Hollingshead, K. W. (2003). *Veterinary Anesthesia and Analgesia* (3rd ed.). St. Louis: Mosby.

Mosley, C. A. (2015). Anesthesia. In: K. A. Grimm, L. A. Lamont, W. J. Tranquilli, S. A. Greene, and S. A. Robertson (Eds.), *Veterinary Anesthesia and Analgesia: The Fifth Edition of Lumb and Jones* (pp. 23–85). Ames: John Wiley & Sons, Inc.

Muir, W. W., Hubbell, J. A., Bednarski, P., and Lerche, P. (2013). *Handbook of Veterinary Anesthesia, 5th edn.* St. Louis: Elsevier Mosby.

Quandt, J. E., Lee, J. A., and Powell, L. L. (2005). Analgesia in critically ill patients. *Compen Contin Educ Prac Vet*, 27(6), 433–445.

Rondeau, M., and Hanie, E. A. (2014). History and physical examination. In J. M. Bassert, and J. A. Thomas, *McCurnin's Clinical Textbook for Veterinary Technicians, 8th edn*, (pp. 221–257). St. Louis: Elsevier Saunders.

Thomas, J. A., and Lerche, P. (2011). *Anesthesia and Analgesia for Veterinary Technicians, 4th edn*. St. Louis: Mosby.

Veterinary Anesthesia and Analgesia Support Group (2015). *Anesthetic Induction Routine* Retrieved from Veterinary Anesthesia and Analgesia Support Group Web Site: www.vasg.org/anesthetic_induction.htm (accessed September 14, 2016).

Wiese, A. J., Muir, W. W., and Wittum, T. E. (2005). Characteristics of pain and response to analgesic treatment in dogs and cats examined at a veterinary teaching hospital emergency service. *J Amer Vet Med Assoc*, 226(12), 2004–2009.

5

Surgical Nursing and Assisting

Laurie J. Buell and Lisa E. Schenkel

5.1 Fundamentals of Common Surgical Procedures

The veterinary technology student is required to have knowledge of the following procedures and pertinent equipment. (AVMA Committee on Veterinary Technician Education and Activities, 2016)

1) **The student displays knowledge of ovariohysterectomy in dogs and cats.**
   - The student correctly explains ovariohysterectomy as the surgical removal of the uterus and ovaries.
   - The student demonstrates knowledge of correct patient preparation and positioning, anesthesia and analgesia, surgical assisting, aftercare, and necessary equipment and instrumentation for ovariohysterectomy in dogs and cats.
   - The student displays understanding of the effects of ovariohysterectomy on the health and behavior of dogs and cats.
   - The student shows awareness of considerations regarding age and the estrous cycle in scheduling ovariohysterectomy in dogs and cats.
   - The student displays knowledge of common complications associated with ovariohysterectomy in dogs and cats.

2) **The student demonstrates knowledge of Cesarean section.**
   - The student correctly explains Cesarean section as removal of the fetus through an incision in the abdominal wall and uterus. Student demonstrates knowledge that Cesarean section is a surgical procedure for dystocia or medical emergency during pregnancy, such as pelvic fracture.
   - The student shows awareness of the breeds that are expected to require Caesarean section, for example, the English Bulldog.
   - The student demonstrates knowledge of correct patient preparation and positioning, anesthesia

and analgesia, surgical assisting, aftercare, and necessary equipment and instrumentation for Cesarean section.
   - The student demonstrates awareness of common complications associated with Caesarian section.
   - The student displays knowledge of how to properly prepare an appropriate environment for the newborns (i.e., a clean, dry area of plenty of towels).
   - The student correctly explains appropriate steps to take to initiate spontaneous respiration and achieve cardiovascular stability in the newborn. The student describes proper procedure for ligating the umbilicus and reuniting the newborn with the mother.

3) **The student displays knowledge of orthopedic procedures.**
   - The student displays awareness of orthopedic procedures as those involving the skeleton, joints, and associated structures.
   - The student shows understanding of orthopedic terms and abbreviations, such as cranial cruciate ligament (CCL), medial patellar luxation (MPL), and intervertebral disk disease (IVDD).
   - The student demonstrates knowledge of correct patient preparation and positioning, anesthesia and analgesia, surgical assisting, aftercare, and necessary equipment and instrumentation for orthopedic procedures.
   - The student displays awareness of the benefits of rehabilitation therapy as part of the post-operative care of the orthopedic patient.

4) **The student displays knowledge of orchiectomy in common species.**
   - The student displays awareness of castration as removal of the testes.
   - The student demonstrates knowledge of correct patient preparation and positioning, anesthesia and analgesia, surgical assisting, aftercare, and necessary equipment and instrumentation for castration.

Assessing Essential Skills of Veterinary Technology Students, Third Edition. Edited by Laurie J. Buell, Lisa E. Schenkel and Sabrina Timperman.
© 2017 John Wiley & Sons, Inc. Published 2017 by John Wiley & Sons, Inc.
Companion website: www.wiley.com/go/buell/skills

- The student displays knowledge of the effects of orchiectomy on the health and behavior of dogs and cats.
- The student shows awareness of considerations regarding age on the scheduling of orchiectomy in dogs and cats.
- The student shows awareness of common complications associated with orchiectomy.

5) **The student displays knowledge of tail docking.**
- The student demonstrates understanding that the term "tail docking" generally refers to the partial amputation of the tail for aesthetic reasons; however, tail amputation may be medically necessary to treat trauma, infection or neoplasia of the tail.
- The student demonstrates knowledge of correct patient preparation and positioning, anesthesia and analgesia, surgical assisting, aftercare, and necessary equipment and instrumentation for tail docking.
- The student displays awareness of the common complications associated with tail docking and tail amputation.

6) **The student displays knowledge of onychectomy in dogs and cats.**
- The student demonstrates awareness of onychectomy in cats as surgical amputation of the third phalanx and claw, and in dogs as surgical removal of the dewclaw.
- The student demonstrates knowledge of correct patient preparation and positioning, anesthesia and analgesia, surgical assisting, aftercare, and necessary equipment and instrumentation for onychectomy.
- The student displays awareness of common complications associated with onychectomy.

7) **The student displays knowledge of laparotomy.**
- The student demonstrates knowledge of general indications for laparotomy in all common species, for example, the presence of abdominal foreign bodies, trauma, gastric dilatation volvulus or abdominal masses.
- The student displays awareness of laparotomy as surgical incision through the abdominal wall.
- The student demonstrates knowledge of correct patient preparation and positioning, anesthesia and analgesia, surgical assisting, aftercare, and necessary equipment and instrumentation for laparotomy.
- The student displays awareness of the common complications associated with laparotomy as well as complications related to specific indications.

8) **The student displays knowledge of dystocia in common species.**
- The student demonstrates awareness of dystocia as difficult birth.
- The student shows knowledge that dystocia is more prevalent in certain breeds, for example, chondrodystrophics.

- The student displays knowledge of normal stages of labor as well as the criteria for dystocia.
- The student shows awareness that dystocia is an emergency situation requiring prompt veterinary intervention.
- The student displays knowledge of potential complications of dystocia.

9) **The student displays knowledge of dehorning in cattle and goats.**
- The student displays knowledge of dehorning as removal of the horns.
- The student displays knowledge of different dehorning techniques used in animals of different ages. For example, when possible, cows should be dehorned with a dehorning iron at less than one month old or when the horn buds are first felt. Beef calves, however, are dehorned at the time of weaning, commonly with a Barnes dehorner or scoop (Mitchell, 2014).
- The student demonstrates knowledge of correct patient preparation and positioning, anesthesia and analgesia, surgical assisting, aftercare, and necessary equipment and instrumentation for dehorning in cattle and goats.
- The student displays recognition that the use of a multimodal approach to analgesia, including the use of a local anesthetic, an anti-inflammatory agent and, when possible, a sedative-analgesic agent, is recommended to diminish the acute phase of pain associated with dehorning (Stock, Baldridge, Griffin et al., 2013).
- The student displays knowledge of potential complications of dehorning.

10) **The student displays knowledge of the correction of prolapsed organs.**
- The student demonstrates awareness of organ prolapse as displacement of the organ. For example, uterine prolapse occurs when the uterus becomes everted so that the cervix is displaced through the vaginal orifice.
- The student displays knowledge of common types of organ prolapse, in which species they occur and how frequently they occur. For example, prolapse of the nictitans gland is the most common disorder affecting the third eyelid in dogs.
- The student demonstrates awareness of the types of organ prolapse that are emergency situations requiring prompt veterinary intervention.
- The student demonstrates knowledge of correct patient preparation and positioning, anesthesia and analgesia, surgical assisting, aftercare, and necessary equipment and instrumentation for correction of various types of organ prolapse.
- The student displays knowledge of potential complications of common types of prolapsed organs.

5.2   Experience with Common Surgical Procedures

The veterinary technology student is required to actively participate in the following procedures. (AVMA Committee on Veterinary Technician Education and Activities, 2016)

11) **The student takes an appropriate active role in the ovariohysterectomy of a dog and a cat.**
   - The student properly prepares all equipment and instrumentation prior to anesthetic induction. The student accurately calculates doses of pre-scribed anesthetic and analgesic agents.
   - The student properly administers prescribed anesthetics and analgesics.
   - The student correctly assists in the procedure, as directed by the veterinarian.
   - The student provides appropriate aftercare for the patient.

12) **The student takes an appropriate active role in the orchiectomy of a dog and a cat.**
   - The student properly prepares all equipment and instrumentation prior to anesthetic induction. The student accurately calculates doses of pre-scribed anesthetic and analgesic agents.
   - The student properly administers prescribed anesthetics and analgesics.
   - The student correctly assists in the procedure, as directed by the veterinarian.
   - The student provides appropriate aftercare for the patient.

5.3   Management of the Veterinary Surgical Patient

13) **The student displays awareness of the need to confirm patient identities, making certain that they correctly match scheduled surgical procedures**
   - The student shows appreciation of the need for diligence in the use of medical records, signal-ment and animal identification methods to make certain that the patient and scheduled surgical procedure correctly match. For example, the patient's name and signalment must be matched to its medical record upon admission to the facil-ity and before every treatment. In addition, the patient's medical problem(s) and reason for sur-gery must be confirmed. The student displays rec-ognition of the importance of properly labeling the patient's cage with all pertinent information.
   - In facilities using ID bands, the student shows awareness that the band must be attached before the animal is taken from the owner and rechecked prior to every procedure and/or treatment.

14) **The student demonstrates understanding of the need to make certain medical records are in order and all necessary consent forms are properly completed and signed prior to patients undergo-ing surgical procedures.**
   - The student displays the ability to correctly organize and make appropriate, legible entries in medical records, using correct spelling, abbre-viations, and format.
   - The student demonstrates appreciation of medical records and consent forms as legal documents.

15) **The student demonstrates the ability to care-fully and knowledgeably review pre-operative assessment.**
   - Prior to and during the pre-anesthetic period, the student displays awareness of how to appropri-ately work with the veterinarian to gather as much information as possible on the patient relevant to anesthesia.
   - The student shows understanding of the need to review the patient's medical records to make certain all pre-procedural tests ordered by the veterinarian have been completed. The student demonstrates awareness that minimum labora-tory evaluation includes complete blood count (CBC), blood chemistries and urinalysis and dis-plays understanding of why each test is necessary. The student displays knowledge of additional diagnostic tests that the veterinarian may order prior to the procedure and the purposes of each, including but not limited to ECG, coagulation tests and/or radiographs.
   - The student demonstrates adequate ability to understand the results of pre-operative evaluation and explain their pertinence to anesthesia and analgesia.

16) **The student demonstrates the ability to correctly assess up-to-the-minute patient status during the peri-anesthetic period.**
   - The student demonstrates the ability to correctly conduct a brief physical examination prior to the procedure, not to replicate veterinarian's prior physical examination, but to obtain vital signs, help determine baseline parameters in the awake animal (which later can be compared with those obtained during and after anesthesia) and aid in the discovery of any acute abnormalities in the period immediately preceding anesthetic induction.
   - The student displays the ability to carefully observe the behavior of the patient prior to the procedure. This is to help detect any behaviors

associated with pain, but is equally important in animals not thought to be experiencing pain, because it allows comparison with the patient's behavior after the procedure. The student shows awareness that deviation from the individual animal's normal behaviors may be evidence of pain (e.g., inability to sleep, anorexia, depression, apprehensiveness, normally friendly animal behaving aggressively or unwilling to interact, lack of grooming in cats, etc.) (Hansen and Hardie, 1993; Hardie, Hansen, and Carroll, 1997; Hellyer and Gaynor, 1998).

- The student displays the ability to distinguish physical or behavioral abnormalities and to effectively and accurately communicate them to the veterinarian.

17) **The student demonstrates the ability to implement an anesthetic protocol in an organized, well-integrated manner.**

- The student displays the ability to work with the veterinarian to plan and coordinate anesthesia, follow the anesthetic plan in a careful, organized manner, and anticipate and be prepared to respond appropriately to the surgeon's and individual patient's needs.

- The student demonstrates awareness that the longer the animal is kept under anesthesia, the greater the risk of complications. In coordinating anesthesia, therefore, the student shows knowledge of how to take all possible steps to minimize time under anesthesia. For example, all equipment and drugs necessary for anesthetic induction, maintenance and recovery should be checked and prepared well in advance of anesthetic induction.

18) **The student correctly locates and safely palpates the urinary bladder.**

- The student displays awareness of the importance of allowing an animal to urinate prior to the procedure, for example, to alleviate discomfort and to avoid interference of a distended bladder with the procedure.

- The student gives the animal adequate opportunity to urinate at an appropriate time prior to anesthetic induction. For example, walking a dog or giving a cat a litter pan.

- The student uses correct technique in locating and safely palpating the bladder.

- The student displays knowledge of risks associated with manual expression of the bladder. For example, even correct manual expression technique can result in hematuria and bladder rupture.

- The student demonstrates knowledge of conditions in which manual bladder expression would

be contraindicated, such as abdominal trauma, urethral obstruction, and cystotomy.

19) **The student uses correct aseptic technique to prepare the skin at the surgical site.**

- The student demonstrates understanding of the need to minimize microbial flora on the skin at the anticipated surgical site in order to decrease the chance of surgical wound contamination.

- The student demonstrates understanding of appropriate uses and relative advantages and disadvantages of different surgical scrubs and topical antiseptic solutions, such as povidone-iodine, chlorhexidine, and 70% isopropyl alcohol.

- The student uses the appropriate clipper blade to complete fur clipping for surgical site preparation. The student properly maintains the clipper and blades and takes care to avoid skin abrasion or clipper burn.

- The student demonstrates understanding that fur removal and preliminary skin scrubbing are performed in the prep area. After properly identifying the approximate incision site, the student cleanly and evenly removes the fur, leaving sufficient margins around the anticipated incision site, and thoroughly vacuums loose fur. While the patient is still in the prep area, the student correctly performs the initial skin cleansing with surgical scrub solution to remove gross contamination, wearing exam gloves and mask. The student carefully moves the patient to the surgical suite, properly connecting the patient to the anesthetic machine and monitoring devices, and positioning the patient appropriately for the procedure. The student performs the final skin scrub, using correct aseptic technique.

20) **The student demonstrates knowledge of standard positions and properly positions patients for routine surgical procedures.**

- When appropriate, the student asks the surgeon for any personal preferences in patient positioning.

- The student positions and secures patients properly in a manner that provides optimal convenience for the surgeon and safety for the patient. The student uses positioning devices appropriately.

- The student makes certain to keep the airway patent at all times and to connect monitoring devices to the patient in a way that does not interfere with patient positioning or have the potential to compromise the sterile field.

- The student adjusts the surgery table height and lights to meet the needs of the surgeon and procedure.

- The student places appropriate barriers between the patient and surgery table, such as warming devices, towels, and so on.

21) **When providing surgical assistance, the student strictly observes proper operating room conduct and aseptic technique.**
   - The student practices proper daily hygiene, including, but not limited to, keeping fingernails clean, smooth and short, and frequently washing hands. The student displays awareness that nail polish is not recommended and jewelry should be removed prior to entering the surgical suite in order to avoid these items inadvertently falling into or otherwise contaminating the surgical field (Shackelford, 2006). The student avoids the use of perfume or other scents because they can be objectionable to others when working in close quarters and have the potential to mask the odors of anesthetic gases (Tear, 2012).
   - The student shows awareness that any person entering the surgical suite must wash their hands thoroughly and wear a cap, mask and clean surgical scrubs or a gown. The student makes certain to wear only clean shoes in the operating room and follows facility protocol regarding the use of shoe covers.
   - The student correctly distinguishes between sterile and non-sterile personnel. When non-sterile, the student pays constant attention to maintaining aseptic technique and displays appropriate operating room conduct, including but not limited to: keeping movement and talking to a minimum; not reaching across or over a sterile field; not moving objects unnecessarily in the suite once surgery begins; moving behind (never in front of) sterile personnel; never passing between two sterile surfaces or objects; keeping the door to the surgical suite closed, and monitoring patients and equipment without interfering with the surgeon or team.
   - When scrubbing in, the student correctly scrubs hands and forearms and dons gowns, gloves, and other sterile attire properly. The student maintains aseptic procedure at all times.
   - When scrubbed in, the student always keeps their hands and arms in front of the body, above the waist and beneath the shoulders, only touches sterile objects, and moves only in ways that prevent self-contamination, including, but not limited to, facing the surgical field at all times and passing other sterile personnel back-to-back.

22) **The student correctly assists with care of exposed tissues and organs.**
   - The student handles tissues gently, demonstrating understanding that great care is necessary to minimize trauma and injury.
   - The student observes strict aseptic technique at all times when caring for exposed tissues and organs.
   - When assisting in retraction, the student carefully and properly positions hand-held retractors, making certain they are well stabilized to prevent slippage.
   - The student displays awareness that exposed tissues and organs must be kept moist to avoid desiccation. The student shows understanding of why lavage (or irrigation) fluids should be sterile, isotonic, and buffered. The student properly prepares sterile irrigation fluids, warming them when appropriate, and correctly supplies them to surgeon.

23) **The student properly passes instruments and supplies.**
   - The student correctly identifies common surgical instruments, knows the appropriate terminology for each and demonstrates knowledge of their proper uses.
   - The student correctly distinguishes sterile instruments and supplies from those that are non-sterile.
   - The student properly passes sterile items to sterile personnel, maintaining strict aseptic technique.

24) **The student displays knowledge of how to correctly operate and care for suction and cautery devices.**
   - The student demonstrates understanding of how to properly set up both suction and cautery devices, checking that they are functioning properly in advance of the procedure.
   - The student shows awareness of how to correctly prepare necessary attachments and parts in advance, anticipating the surgeon's needs.
   - The student demonstrates familiarity with how to operate suction and cautery devices.
   - The student displays knowledge of the proper cleaning, disinfection and/or sterilization of the various parts of suction and cautery devices.
   - The student shows awareness of safety concerns associated with the use of cautery and suction devices, as well as steps necessary to minimize risks.

25) **The student demonstrates knowledge of principles of operation and proper care of fiber optic equipment.**
   - The student demonstrates familiarity with the difference between flexible and rigid scopes. The student shows awareness that flexible scopes generally are used for gastrointestinal endoscopy, bronchoscopy, and laparoscopy, while rigid scopes are used for such procedures as cystoscopy.
   - The student shows understanding of the basic set-up of the fiber optic unit, including scopes, camera, and computer software. The student displays awareness of the need to handle the equipment with appropriate care.

- The student displays knowledge of the proper care and cleaning of the scope, based on the manufacturer's instruction manual. The student shows awareness that gloves should be worn while cleaning scopes.
- The student recognizes the importance of sterilizing the equipment after use, as well as checking all seals and performing a leak test prior to use. The student shows awareness of the correct procedure for cold sterilization, including thorough rinsing and air drying. The student demonstrates knowledge that personnel should wear gloves (double gloves or frequent glove changes may be recommended) and consult Safety Data Sheets (SDS) prior to using cold sterilization solutions (Lichtenbarger, 2005).
- The student displays knowledge of proper patient preparation for endoscopic procedures.
- The student demonstrates understanding of potential complications associated with fiber optic procedures.

26) **The student maintains thorough, accurate anesthetic/surgical logs.**
- The student displays understanding of the purposes of anesthetic and surgical records.
- The student demonstrates understanding of the importance of maintaining an anesthetic record for each patient, both as legal documentation of significant events and to facilitate identification of trends in monitored values, thereby allowing early recognition of potential complications.
- The student displays understanding of the importance of maintaining a surgical record for each patient, both as legal documentation and to provide data for future analysis (Bassert, 2014).
- The student accurately determines and records all required information in a timely manner. Such information may include, but is not limited to: date, names of surgeon and technician/technologist; names of client and patient; name of procedure; patient signalment; pre-operative, anesthetic, and analgesic agents administered; times administered; dosages administered; percentages of anesthetic gases administered over the surgical period; fluid therapy administered; patient's temperature, heart rate, pulse rate, blood pressure, and respiratory rate over the surgical period; patient's SpO_2 and $ETCO_2$ (and/or blood gases) over the surgical period; manual or mechanical ventilations administered; and the length of pre-anesthesia, anesthesia, and recovery time.

27) **The student demonstrates the ability to coordinate analgesic therapy with members of anesthesia/surgical team.**

- The student displays clear understanding of the roles of each member of the anesthesia/surgical team, including the role of each, if any, in administering analgesic agents and monitoring the individual patient for signs of pain and/or nociception.
- At all times, the student demonstrates appreciation of the need to be certain to keep abreast of any analgesic agents prescribed for and/or administered to the patient during the peri-anesthetic period, including but not limited to, the names of drugs, doses, routes and times of administration, potential drug interactions and the individual patient's response to analgesic agents, including adverse effects.
- When appropriate to the student's role in assessing efficacy of pain management, the student demonstrates understanding of how to be diligent in monitoring the individual patient for evidence of pain and/or nociception throughout the entire perioperative period.
- The student demonstrates awareness of the importance of closely monitoring patients for common adverse responses to various analgesic agents and immediately notifying the supervisor/veterinarian.

28) **The student displays understanding of current methods of pain management in the perioperative patient.**
- The student displays the ability to properly administer analgesic agents, as prescribed by the veterinarian, while continuing to monitor the patient's ongoing status.
- Given that no universally accepted system for classifying and measuring pain intensity in animals yet exists, accurate, objective assessment of the pain intensity experienced by animals can present significant challenges even for experienced veterinarians and veterinary technologists/technicians. In view of this difficulty, the student is appreciative of the need to be diligent in monitoring and displays the ability to assess pain levels as well as to assess the efficacy of pain therapy in the individual animal.
- The student demonstrates basic understanding of appropriate uses, major contraindications, common adverse effects, and appropriate routes and methods of administration for commonly used analgesic agents. These may include, but are not limited to, opioid analgesic agents (and their reversal agents), non-steroidal anti-inflammatory agents, NMDA-receptor antagonists (such as ketamine), and local anesthetic agents.
- The student displays the ability to accurately calculate doses/dosages of common analgesic agents,

including those administered as boluses and those administered as constant rate infusions (CRIs).

- The student exhibits awareness of non-pharmacologic approaches to pain, such as ice compresses, massage and passive range of motion, as well as their appropriate uses.

29) **The student indicates understanding of the principles of fluid therapy in the perioperative period, based on the needs of the individual patient.**

- The student displays the ability to accurately calculate fluid infusion rates, based on the veterinarian's orders. The student shows the ability to administer intravenous fluids at proper rates, correctly operating infusion pumps and various fluid delivery systems.
- The student shows awareness of the need to frequently monitor fluid administration to ensure that the fluid is flowing freely at the correct rate and demonstrates the ability to make appropriate corrections or adjustments, when necessary.
- The student demonstrates the ability to correctly and closely monitor the hydration status of patients. The student exhibits awareness of the potential risks associated with both dehydration and over-hydration.
- The student displays knowledge of various crystalloid solutions, including which are balanced versus non-balanced solutions and which are isotonic, hypotonic, or hypertonic. The student shows awareness of proper indications and major contraindications for various types of crystalloid solutions, as well as any special requirements for their administration.
- The student displays knowledge of various colloids, including natural and synthetic, their proper indications and any special requirements for their administration.

30) **The student demonstrates understanding of how to provide adequate nutrition for patients during the postoperative period.**

- The student displays knowledge of various types of diets and shows the ability to select appropriate diets for individual patients.
- The student demonstrates the ability to accurately calculate caloric requirements for selected patients and shows the ability to determine whether or not patients are receiving adequate nutrition and adjust feedings, if necessary.
- The student demonstrates the ability to properly syringe-feed and tube-feed anorexic patients. The student shows awareness of potential risks associated with syringe-feeding and tube-feeding.
- The student demonstrates understanding of potentially dire consequences of inadequate nutrition in

animals, including but not limited to hepatic lipidosis in cats, decreased hepatic protein synthesis, and so on.
- The student displays familiarity with the use of parental nutrition in anorexic patients.

31) **The student demonstrates understanding of how to properly care for wounds during the post-procedural period.**

- The student displays knowledge of wound classification and the principles of wound healing.
- The student shows knowledge of proper wound care based on a familiarity with post-operative wound closure techniques, such as suturing and stapling.
- The student displays awareness of the need to protect wounds from mutilation through use of Elizabethan collars, and so on.
- The student demonstrates the ability to recognize signs of wound infection (i.e., swelling, redness, exudate, odor, etc.) and wound closure failure. In addition, the student shows the ability to identify the need for treatment and to inform the supervisor and/or veterinarian.
- The student exhibits the ability to properly explain to clients proper wound care techniques and what signs may indicate infection and/or other problems.

32) **The student displays understanding of how to properly care for bandages during the post-procedural period.**

- The student demonstrates knowledge of various bandages and shows the ability to select the type of bandage appropriate for the specific surgical procedure and the individual patient.
- The student displays the ability to choose an appropriate primary (contact) layer based on the wound or operative site and to apply primary, secondary, and tertiary layers of the bandage correctly.
- The student shows knowledge of proper bandage care and of when to change a bandage, displaying awareness of how to closely monitor the bandage for slippage, wetness, soiling, signs of excessive tightness (e.g., toe swelling), and so on.
- The student demonstrates the ability to recognize an inappropriately applied bandage or a failed bandage.

33) **The student demonstrates the ability to provide understandable, accurate discharge instructions to the client in a manner that maximizes likelihood of compliance.**

- The student displays adequate understanding of the procedures performed in order to accurately and effectively communicate discharge instructions to the client.

- The student shows the ability to explain, in a manner that is clear and understandable to most clients, proper wound care, how to monitor sutures and/or the surgical site (i.e., for signs of infection or closure failure), proper bandage care (including how to recognize a failed or excessively tight bandage), proper application and care of Elizabethan collars, directions for administering prescribed drugs, appropriate activity levels for the patient, appropriate feeding techniques and specialized diets for post-operative patients, and so on.
- The student demonstrates the ability to explain to clients, in an understandable, courteous, and tactful manner, the importance of compliance with discharge instructions.
- The student displays the ability to explain the need for follow-up appointments in a manner that maximizes the likelihood of compliance.

34) **The student removes sutures in a safe and correct manner.**
- The student properly distinguishes between absorbable and non-absorbable suture material. The student displays familiarity with the use of intradermal sutures for wound closure and shows awareness that, although they do not require removal, the wound should be monitored and rechecked for proper healing.
- The student shows the ability to recognize signs of suture failure (i.e., dehiscence) or damage.
- Based on the veterinarian's instructions, the student displays the ability to accurately determine the appropriate time period for suture removal.
- The student displays the ability to recognize adequate wound healing prior to removing sutures.
- When removing sutures, the student shows the ability to determine the best site at which to cut the suture, (i.e., that which will minimize the length of suture being brought back through the body). The student safely and correctly removes sutures and staples.

5.4 Management of Surgical Equipment and Facilities

35) **The student correctly prepares instruments, instrument packs, and surgical supplies.**
- The student demonstrates familiarity with common surgical instruments and knowledge of the correct terminology for each.
- The student displays knowledge of instruments required for common surgical procedures and correctly prepares instrument packs for various common surgical procedures.

- Prior to sterilization, the student checks each instrument to make certain it is completely clean, lubricated (e.g., in instrument milk) when appropriate, in good repair and properly functioning.
- The student demonstrates knowledge of appropriate wrap materials and makes certain wraps are clean, dry, and in good condition, without tears or holes.
- The student correctly assembles packs, checking that they are complete, properly and tightly wrapped, contain a dependable sterilization indicator, and are taped closed and labeled properly.
- The student makes certain surgical packs, supplies, and equipment are sterilized and ready for use in advance of procedures.
- The student properly stores instruments to maintain sterility and makes certain they are ready for the next procedure.
- The student displays knowledge of circumstances in which sterility is compromised, including but not limited to, penetration of moisture, tears, punctures, breakage of seals, excessive handling, exceeding shelf life, and so on (Caveney, 2006; Tear, 2012).
- The student demonstrates the ability to anticipate the surgical team's needs, to assemble instruments and supplies required for common procedures, and to prepare the surgical suite correctly. The student furnishes the correct items in a timely manner, when requested by the surgical team.

36) **The student correctly prepares gowns, masks, gloves, and drapes.**
- The student displays familiarity with different types of gowns and gown materials, types of masks, gloves, head covers, and protective footwear.
- The student lays out appropriate types and sizes of surgical gloves for the surgical team. The student displays the ability to assist the surgeon in gowning.
- If reusable gowns and drapes are used, the student correctly washes, dries and folds gowns and drapes after use. The student correctly assembles packs containing gowns or drapes, folding them properly, using appropriate wrap materials, enclosing dependable sterilization indicators, taping them closed and labeling them properly.
- The student correctly differentiates closed gloving from open gloving, and displays the ability to assist the surgeon in changing gloves during procedure.
- The student demonstrates the ability to correctly scrub-in and join the sterile surgical team by: donning a mask, cap and shoe covers; performing a sterile scrub; donning a surgical gown, and performing closed and open gloving.

37) The student safely operates and properly cares for autoclaves.

- The student displays awareness of different sizes and types of autoclaves.
- The student demonstrates understanding of the autoclaving process and how it produces sterilization, when functioning properly.
- The student correctly and safely operates the autoclave according to the manufacturer's recommendations, filling it with distilled water to the appropriate level, determining the proper time, temperature and pressure requirements to sterilize each instrument and/or pack and properly loading it for optimal performance.
- The student displays familiarity with various types of packaging material and selects the appropriate type for each item.
- The student properly determines when the autoclaving cycle is complete and vents the autoclave at the correct time.
- The student safely removes items from the autoclave.
- The student displays knowledge of the various types of sterilization indicators and the proper use of each.
- The student stores sterilized instruments, packs and supplies appropriately.

38) The student correctly differentiates disinfection from sterilization and properly utilizes various methods of disinfection and sterilization.

- The student displays awareness that sterilization destroys all microorganisms and pathogenic matter on inanimate objects, while disinfection destroys or inhibits growth of most microorganisms and pathogenic matter on inanimate objects.
- The student shows understanding that cold sterilization involves immersion of an object in a disinfectant solution, and may be used to achieve different levels of disinfection, depending upon the concentration used and the contact time (Caveney, 2006).
- The student properly utilizes agents such as glutaraldehyde and benzalkonium chloride solutions for cold sterilization. The student wears gloves when preparing or touching cold sterilization solutions.
- The student safely and properly utilizes various sterilization methods, including autoclaving and gas sterilization (e.g., ethylene oxide and/or gas plasma). The student displays knowledge of potential hazards associated with ethylene oxide sterilization as well as limitations of gas sterilization methods.

- The student demonstrates awareness that cold sterilization is appropriate only in limited circumstances, such as disinfection of instruments or equipment that would be damaged by other means of sterilization.
- The student demonstrates knowledge of procedures requiring sterilized instruments, for example, those in which an instrument touches tissues under the skin (Shackelford, 2006).

39) The student correctly and efficiently sets up all needed instrumentation and equipment prior to the surgical procedure.

- The student demonstrates knowledge of all instrumentation and equipment necessary for common surgical procedures.
- The student checks all instruments and equipment in advance of the procedure to ensure it is in proper working order.
- The student handles all instrumentation and equipment properly, maintaining aseptic technique when appropriate.
- The student makes certain that surgical set-up is completed prior to anesthetic induction to minimize the patient's time under anesthesia.

40) The student demonstrates knowledge of the correct names and proper uses of commonly used instruments.

- The student correctly identifies specific surgical instruments and groups them into such categories as scalpel blades, scalpel handles, scissors, hemostats, needle holders, towel clamps, forceps, retractors (hand-held and self-retaining), orthopedic instruments, and so on.
- The student displays understanding of appropriate uses of specific, commonly used instruments. For example, Kelly forceps are hemostats used to crush blood vessels, Metzenbaum scissors are used to cut delicate tissues, Backhaus towel clamps are used to secure drapes to the patient, and so on.
- The student displays knowledge of the instruments that are likely to be required for common surgical procedures and which instruments should be included in specific, multi-instrument packs.

41) The student displays the ability to accurately identify types and sizes of suture materials and needles.

- The student demonstrates the ability to differentiate between monofilament and braided, absorbable and non-absorbable and synthetic and natural suture materials.
- The student recognizes both generic and common brand names for suture materials.

- The student displays understanding of conventions for sizing the diameter of suture material, particularly for suture sized below 1. For example, a 2-0 suture has a smaller diameter than a 1-0 suture, and a 1-0 suture has a smaller diameter than 0.
- The student properly distinguishes between swaged needles and eyed needles.
- The student shows knowledge of commonly used types and sizes of suture needles, including but not limited to cutting, taper, reverse cutting, and so on.
- The student demonstrates familiarity with common uses of various types of suture needles and suture materials.

42) **The student properly cleans and maintains the operating room.**

- The student demonstrates knowledge of effective cleaning protocols and uses detergent/disinfectant solutions appropriate for cleaning specific surfaces or objects. The student displays knowledge of the amount of contact time necessary for each type to achieve effective disinfection.
- The student damp wipes all horizontal surfaces before the first surgery of the day to minimize airborne contaminants. The student cleans the operating room at the end of each procedure, prior to the entry of the next patient (Tear, 2012). At the end of every day, even when the operating room has not been used, the student cleans all surfaces (including the floor) and equipment with disinfectant solution, taking care to wipe lights (to prevent dust from falling onto the sterile field).
- The student demonstrates awareness that, at least once a week, all equipment and supplies should be removed from the operating room and all surfaces, including floors, walls, doors, door handles, wheels, foot pedals, lights, and so on, scrubbed with an appropriate detergent/disinfectant solution. All equipment also should be cleaned with an appropriate detergent/disinfectant solution.
- The student keeps cleaning implements and buckets designated for operating room use only separated from other cleaning equipment. To minimize microbial contamination, the student makes certain that cleaning implements and buckets are thoroughly washed, rinsed, and allowed to dry prior to being stored.

43) **The student displays knowledge of how to properly maintain aseptic technique in the operating room.**

- The student demonstrates appreciation of the importance of keeping the surgical area as free of microorganisms as possible.

- The student accurately demarcates the entire sterile field.
- The student shows understanding of proper operating room conduct. For example, sterile personnel should only touch sterile items and non-sterile personnel should only touch non-sterile items.
- The student demonstrates knowledge of how to correctly introduce items into a sterile field while maintaining sterility; for example, how to properly open wraps and pouches, how to appropriately transfer instruments and how to correctly pour irrigation fluids.
- The student displays understanding of how to move in a manner that maintains the integrity of the sterile field. The student shows awareness that movement should be minimized to decrease air currents that could contaminate the sterile field.
- The student shows appreciation of the importance of restricting conversation and keeping the door to the operating room closed as much as possible.
- The student displays understanding of the importance of immediately reporting and correcting any violation of aseptic technique (Tear, 2012).

44) **The student properly cleans the operating room following surgical procedures.**

- The student safely removes scalpel blades from handles and properly deposits scalpel blades and needles in appropriate sharps containers.
- The student correctly disposes of used paper items, such as drapes, gauze sponges, masks, disposable gowns, and so on.
- The student places all used cloth items, such as towels, drapes, gowns, and so on, into detergent solution to pre-soak. The student demonstrates knowledge that surgical items should be laundered separately from all other laundry.
- The student makes certain to confirm with the surgeon which tissues, organs or other organic material must be kept for laboratory analysis, and handles, labels, stores, and packages them appropriately.
- The student properly disposes of hazardous medical waste.
- The student carefully and safely removes instruments and packs from the operating room. The student removes organic material such as blood or tissue from instruments as soon as possible to prevent pitting and/or corrosion, pre-soaking them in an appropriate instrument cleaning solution. Making certain that box locks and ratchets are open, the student correctly and thoroughly cleans, rinses, lubricates (when appropriate), and dries instruments. The student checks each

instrument to make certain it is in good repair and functioning properly.
- The student makes certain to shut off warming and monitoring devices, gas cylinders and lines, cautery and suction equipment and scavenging systems.

- The student soaks rebreathing bags, anesthetic hoses, and so on in appropriate disinfectant solution, rinses them thoroughly and hangs them to dry completely prior to use.
- The student correctly cleans the operating room after each procedure.

References

Bassert, J. M. (2014). Veterinary medical records. In: J. M. Bassert, and J. A. Thomas, *McCurnin's Clinical Textbook for Veterinary Technicians*, 8th edn (pp. 80–113). St. Louis: Elsevier Saunders.

Committee on Veterinary Technician Education and Activities (2016). Accreditation Policies and Procedures of the AVMA Committee on Veterinary Technician Education and Activities (CVTEA). Retrieved June 2, 2016 from www.avma.org/ProfessionalDevelopment/Education/Accreditation/Programs/Pages/cvtea-pp-appendix-i.aspx (accessed September 14, 2016).

Caveney, L. M. (2006). Cleaning, disinfection and sterilization procedures. *Vet Tech*, 27(4), 236–240.

Lichtenbarger, M. (2005). Gastrointestinal endoscopy: procedures and equipment care. *Vet Tech*, 26(6), 404–416.

Mitchell, C. F. (2014). Large animal surgical nursing. In: J. M. Bassert, and J. A. Thomas, *Technicians, McCurnin's Clinical Textbook for Veterinary*, 8th edn (pp. 1259–1296). St. Louis: Elsevier Saunders.

Shackelford, S. (2006). Aseptic technique for surgery. *Veterinary Technician*, 25(1), pp. 49–52.

Stock, M. L., Baldridge, S. L., Griffin, D., et al. (2013, March). Bovine dehorning: assessing pain and providing analgesic management. *Vet Clin North Am Food Anim Pract*, 29(1), 103–133.

Tear, M. (2012). *Small Animal Surgical Nursing Skills and Concepts*, 2nd edn. St. Louis: Elsevier Mosby.

6

Clinical Laboratory Procedures

Lisa E. Schenkel, Sabrina Timperman, Laurie J. Buell, Judy Duffelmeyer-Kramer,
Robin E. Sturtz and Deirdre Douglas

6.1 Management of Laboratory Specimens and Equipment

1) **The student properly chooses and cares for laboratory equipment.**
   - The student describes the functions of common pieces of laboratory equipment. Based on this understanding, the student correctly chooses equipment for the requested test procedure.
   - The student displays awareness of the importance of organizing and storing equipment-use manuals.
   - The student properly cleans common laboratory equipment according to manufacturers' recommendations.

2) **The student participates in employing quality control procedures.**
   - The student shows understanding of the importance of quality control in achieving accurate results.
   - The student displays understanding of the importance of maintenance logs and uses them appropriately.
   - The student participates in performing calibration of common laboratory equipment according to manufacturers' recommendations.
   - The student demonstrates the ability to differentiate accurate from incorrect results, considering the individual patient as well as specimen submitted.

3) **The student demonstrates understanding of how to take all necessary steps to maximize the safety of patients, clients, and staff.**
   - The student demonstrates knowledge of appropriate laboratory conduct.
   - The student demonstrates knowledge of the locations of safety features of a laboratory, such as SDS, fire emergency equipment, emergency exits, eye wash stations and showers, emergency exit maps, and so on. The student displays the ability to appropriately utilize laboratory safety features.
   - The student evidences awareness of potential safety hazards and carries out laboratory procedures without breaking safety protocols.
   - The student describes the appropriate use of personal protective equipment in the laboratory.
   - The student displays appreciation of the importance of rigorous hygiene, thoroughly washing hands, wearing gloves when appropriate and cleaning all work areas with suitable disinfectants after use.
   - The student makes certain that no food or beverages are permitted in laboratory areas.
   - The student appropriately disposes of sharps into sharps containers and biohazard materials into biohazard bags/containers.

4) **The student correctly prepares, labels, packages, and stores samples for diagnostic laboratory examination.**
   - The student prepares and processes laboratory samples appropriately based on a correct understanding of the use of such samples in diagnostic tests.
   - The student demonstrates precise labelling of diagnostic samples.
   - The student handles, packages and stores diagnostic samples in a manner that ensures the maximum accuracy of results.

6.2 Diagnostic Laboratory Procedures

5) **The student correctly determines the physical properties of urine samples.**
   - The student accurately describes the color, clarity and odor of the sample, using appropriate terminology.

Assessing Essential Skills of Veterinary Technology Students, Third Edition. Edited by Laurie J. Buell, Lisa E. Schenkel and Sabrina Timperman.
© 2017 John Wiley & Sons, Inc. Published 2017 by John Wiley & Sons, Inc.
Companion website: www.wiley.com/go/buell/skills

- The student correctly defines and displays understanding of the diagnostic significance of urine specific gravity. The student properly uses the refractometer to measure the urine specific gravity, cleaning it properly after each use. The student frequently checks the calibration of the refractometer and correctly recalibrates it as needed.

- The student demonstrates understanding of reagent strips used to determine the chemical properties of urine. The student uses reagent strips properly, reading results accurately. The student evidences awareness that, depending on the species being tested, false positive and false negative results regarding the presence of cellular elements in urine may occur; therefore, these results should be verified with microscopic sediment analysis.

- The student describes the significance of the color, clarity, odor, and specific gravity of the urine sample as they relate to the clinical condition.

- The student properly prepares urine sediment for microscopic examination. Using correct microscopic technique, the student accurately identifies red blood cells, white blood cells, crystals, casts, artifacts, and so on, using experience and reference books.

- The student explains the significance of the results of the microscopic analysis as they relate to the clinical condition.

6) **The student demonstrates knowledge of how to accurately determine the hemoglobin concentration of a complete blood count (CBC).**

- The student correctly explains the difference between plasma and serum.

- The student correctly defines the term "hemoglobin," and correctly describes the physiological functions of hemoglobin and the clinical relevance of the hemoglobin concentration.

- The student displays knowledge of the appropriate blood sample tube and anticoagulant for obtaining an accurate hemoglobin concentration.

- The student demonstrates the ability to accurately calculate the hemoglobin concentration.

7) **The student demonstrates correct methodology for obtaining a packed cell volume (PCV).**

- The student correctly explains the difference between plasma and serum.

- The student correctly defines the term "packed cell volume" and correctly explains its clinical relevance.

- The student displays awareness that, although the terms PCV and hematocrit (HCT) often are used interchangeably in the clinical setting, the HCT is a value calculated by automatic analyzers whereas the PCV is directly measured manually.

- The student uses the appropriate blood sample tube and anticoagulant for obtaining an accurate HCT.

- The student demonstrates the proper use of the microhematocrit tube and centrifuge to obtain a PCV.

- The student observes and makes note of the characteristics of the plasma, including color and turbidity.

- The student correctly measures the PCV.

8) **The student demonstrates correct methodology for determining the total protein concentration.**

- The student correctly explains the difference between plasma and serum.

- The student correctly explains the difference in the major protein constituents of plasma versus serum and describes the physiological functions and clinical relevance of each.

- The student uses the appropriate blood sample tube and anticoagulant to obtain the total protein concentration.

- The student demonstrates the proper use of the microhematocrit tube and centrifuge to obtain the total protein concentration.

- The student observes and makes note of the characteristics of the plasma, including color and turbidity.

- The student properly uses a refractometer to obtain the total protein concentration.

9) **The student demonstrates correct methodology for obtaining a white blood cell count.**

- The student correctly explains the difference between plasma and serum.

- The student correctly describes the general physiological functions of white blood cells and the clinical relevance of a white blood cell count.

- The student correctly identifies the constituents of a buffy coat.

- The student uses the appropriate blood sample tube and anticoagulant for obtaining a white blood cell count.

- The student demonstrates proper use of the microhematocrit tube and centrifuge to obtain the buffy coat.

- The student observes and makes note of the characteristics of the buffy coat.

- The student accurately determines the white blood cell count.

10) **The student demonstrates correct methodology for obtaining a red blood cell count.**

- The student correctly explains the difference between plasma and serum.

- The student correctly describes the general physiological functions of red blood cells and clinical relevance of a red blood cell count.
- The student correctly explains the difference between the PCV and the red blood cell count.
- The student uses the appropriate blood sample tube and anticoagulant for obtaining a red blood cell count.
- The student accurately determines the red blood cell count.

11) **The student uses proper methodology to prepare blood films, showing proficiency in staining them with a variety of techniques.**
   - The student correctly prepares blood smears of appropriate length, width, and density
   - The student shows familiarity with various stains and their appropriate applications.
   - The student uses proper technique to stain blood films.

12) **The student demonstrates correct methodology for performing a leukocyte differential and accurately distinguishes between normal and abnormal cells.**
   - The student evaluates the condition and state of all cells on the blood smear.
   - The student accurately identifies types of leukocytes.
   - The student accurately differentiates between normal and abnormal cells and correctly explains the clinical relevance of commonly seen morphological changes.
   - The student performs a count of 100 leukocytes for the differential and accurately determines relative counts for each white cell type.
   - The student displays understanding of the clinical significance of abnormal counts of each type of leukocyte.

13) **The student correctly assesses the morphology of erythrocytes and accurately distinguishes between normal and abnormal cells.**
   - The student correctly evaluates red blood cells for morphological differences, demonstrating understanding of species differences. The student accurately identifies rouleaux formation, spherocytes, poikilocytes, macrocytes, microcytes, anisocytosis, polychromasia, and so on.
   - The student accurately differentiates between normal and abnormal cells, and distinguishes changes due to disease from those due to artifact or mechanical causes. The student correctly observes inclusions such as Howell–Jolly bodies and Heinz bodies, as well as parasites, such as *Babesia* spp. and *Hemobartonella* spp.
   - The student demonstrates understanding of the diagnostic importance of erythrocyte morphology.

14) **The student demonstrates correct methodology for estimating thrombocyte numbers.**
   - The student correctly describes some of the species differences in platelet counts and appearance, as well as how these species differences affect the ability to obtain an accurate platelet count.
   - The student utilizes proper technique to perform estimated platelet counts on blood films.
   - The student accurately calculates estimated total platelet counts.
   - The student displays knowledge of the diagnostic importance of platelet counts.

15) **The student accurately determines absolute values of leukocytes.**
   - The student accurately calculates absolute values of leukocytes based on the relative percentages and total white blood cell count.
   - The student demonstrates understanding of the diagnostic significance of absolute values of leukocytes.

16) **The student demonstrates proper methodology for performing corrected white blood cell counts due to the presence of other nucleated cells.**
   - The student explains the clinical significance of the presence of other nucleated cells in various species. For example, the nucleated red blood cell is normal in birds. In dogs and cats, however, the presence of nucleated red blood cells is abnormal and may be clinically significant.
   - The student demonstrates understanding of the necessity for performing a corrected white blood cell count due to the presence of other nucleated cells.
   - The student accurately calculates the corrected white blood cell count.

17) **The student correctly determines red blood cell indices.**
   - The student demonstrates knowledge of the diagnostic meaning of red blood cell indices, including MCV, MCH, MCHC, and reticulocyte count.
   - The student demonstrates correct methodology for performing a reticulocyte count by counting 1000 red blood cells and accurately determining the relative percentage of reticulocytes.
   - The student demonstrates an understanding that reticulocyte counts should be interpreted in light of the degree of anemia present and accurately calculates a corrected reticulocyte count.
   - The student correctly calculates MCV.
   - The student correctly differentiates normal versus abnormal values for RBC indices and explains the clinical significance of abnormalities.

18) **The student participates in correctly performing at least one of the following tests of blood coagulation: buccal mucosal bleeding time, activated clotting time (ACT), prothrombin time (PT), partial thromboplastin time (PTT), or fibrinogen assay.**
   - The student demonstrates knowledge of the diagnostic significance of blood coagulation tests (e.g., buccal mucosal bleeding time is used to assess primary hemostasis).
   - The student explains the proper procedure for performing the blood coagulation test in which they were participating.
   - The student accurately differentiates between normal versus abnormal results and correctly explains the clinical significance of abnormal results.

19) **The student demonstrates correct methodology for performing blood chemistry tests, including but not limited to, urea nitrogen, glucose, and common enzymes.**
   - The student correctly describes the difference between plasma and serum and explains why blood chemistry tests are performed on serum.
   - The student demonstrates understanding of the diagnostic significance of common blood chemistry tests.
   - The student correctly performs blood chemistry tests.
   - The student accurately differentiates between normal and abnormal results and explains the clinical significance of abnormal results.

20) **The student demonstrates correct methodology for performing serologic assays, including ELISA and slide/card agglutination tests.**
   - The student demonstrates understanding of immunological principles underlying serological tests.
   - The student shows understanding of the diagnostic importance of serological tests
   - The student properly performs and correctly interprets snap tests.
   - The student properly performs and correctly interprets slide/card agglutination tests.

21) **The student accurately identifies adult and immature stages of *Dirofilaria* spp. and *Acanthocheilonema* spp. (formerly *Dipetalonema* spp.).**
   - The student correctly describes the heartworm life cycle.
   - The student accurately differentiates microfilaria of *Dirofilaria* spp. from *Acanthocheilonema* spp. (formerly *Dipetalonema* spp.).
   - The student demonstrates understanding of the clinical significance of the presence of *Dirofilaria* versus *Acanthocheilonema*.

22) **The student correctly identifies *Hemotropic Mycoplasma* spp. (*Hemoplasmas*), formerly *Haemobartonella* spp. and *Eperythrozoon* spp.**
   - The student accurately differentiates blood cell parasites from stain precipitate and artifacts.
   - The student correctly identifies the *Hemotropic Mycoplasma* spp.
   - The student demonstrates understanding of the clinical significance of *Hemotropic Mycoplasma* infection.

23) **The student displays knowledge of how to detect the presence of mites and correctly identifies mites.**
   - The student demonstrates knowledge of the clinical signs of different types of mite infestations and the clinical significance of each.
   - The student shows knowledge of the zoonotic potential of mite infestation.
   - The student displays knowledge of the proper procedure for detecting the presence of ear mites, including how to correctly take the sample from the ear and prepare the slide for microscopic examination.
   - The student demonstrates knowledge of the proper procedure for detecting mites that burrow into the skin, including the correct skin scrape techniques for *Sarcoptes* versus *Demodex* spp. The student shows knowledge of how to prepare the slide for microscopic evaluation. The student accurately identifies *Sarcoptes* and *Demodex* mites.
   - The student shows awareness of how to detect *Sarcoptes* mites or ova in fecal flotation.
   - The student demonstrates knowledge of how to detect the presence of mites living on the skin surface or hair, such as *Cheyletiella*, using a fine-tooth flea comb and/or cellophane tape methods. The student shows knowledge of how to correctly prepare the slide for microscopic examination. The student accurately identifies *Cheyletiella*.

24) **The student displays knowledge of the proper procedure to detect the presence of lice and correctly identifies lice.**
   - The student demonstrates familiarity with life cycle of lice and differentiates between chewing (biting) versus sucking lice.
   - The student shows awareness of routes of transmission (direct contact, fomites) and clinical signs of lice infestation.
   - The student demonstrates knowledge of the proper procedure for detecting the presence of adult or nymphal lice and/or nits, including how to correctly collect nymphal/adult lice and/or nits. The student shows knowledge of how to prepare the slide for microscopic examination. The student accurately identifies lice.

25) **The student displays knowledge of the proper procedure to detect the presence of ticks and correctly identifies ticks.**
   - The student shows knowledge of the basic tick structure (body parts).
   - The student demonstrates knowledge of the role of ticks in carrying and transmitting disease.
   - The student correctly identifies species of ticks acting as vectors for common infectious diseases, including, but not limited to: *Ixodes* spp. (*Borrelia burgdorferi*, Lyme Disease), *Rhipicephalus sanguineous* (babesiosis, ehrlichiosis), *Dermacentor andersoni*, and *Dermacentor variabilis* (Rocky Mountain Spotted Fever), and so on.
   - The student shows knowledge of how to properly inspect an animal for the presence of ticks, including those that may be hidden. The student demonstrates knowledge of how to correctly remove and dispose of ticks.

26) **The student displays knowledge of the proper procedures to detect the presence of fleas and correctly identifies fleas.**
   - The student correctly identifies fleas, including, but not limited to *Ctenocephalides felis*, and shows knowledge of their life cycles.
   - The student shows knowledge of the role of fleas in carrying and transmitting infectious disease, such as *Dipylidium caninum*.
   - The student demonstrates knowledge of the common clinical signs of flea infestation and flea allergy dermatitis.
   - The student displays knowledge of how to properly inspect an animal for the presence of fleas and/or flea dirt.

27) **The student displays knowledge of the proper procedures to detect the presence of flies and correctly identifies flies.**
   - The student correctly identifies flies and shows familiarity with their life cycles.
   - The student shows knowledge of common clinical signs of fly bites as well as clinical signs of fly larvae that invade the body. The student demonstrates cognizance of the role of flies as vectors for infectious disease.
   - The student accurately identifies maggot infestation.
   - The student shows knowledge that a skin lesion with a central pore is a sign of *Cuterebra* infestation.

28) **The student uses correct methodology to perform heartworm diagnostic procedures, including the antigen kit, direct (examination of blood), and the modified Knotts test.**
   - The student displays knowledge of the immunological basis of the heartworm antigen test.
   - The student shows cognizance of the potential for false negative results on the antigen test and why they occur.
   - The student demonstrates knowledge of the importance of timing the antigen kit test based on the heartworm life cycle in order to maximize accuracy of results.
   - The student properly performs and accurately interprets the results of the heartworm antigen test kit.
   - The student displays knowledge of how to detect microfilaria by observing their movement beneath the buffy coat in a microhematocrit tube or during microscopic examination of a drop of blood.
   - The student demonstrates knowledge of the reasons why a modified Knotts test is the preferred method for identifying microfilaria (American Heartworm Society, 2014a,b).
   - The student participates in properly performing a modified Knotts test.
   - The student accurately identifies *Dirofilaria* microfilaria.
   - The student shows familiarity with the American Heartworm Society's guidelines for heartworm disease testing (American Heartworm Society, 2014a,b).

29) **The student uses correct methodology to perform fecal flotation tests to detect presence of internal parasites.**
   - The student demonstrates understanding of the need for the solution to have a higher specific gravity than parasite ova or larvae in order for the parasitic material to float.
   - The student displays knowledge of the flotation method for concentrating internal parasites. The student shows familiarity with appropriate uses of common flotation solutions, including, but not limited to, sodium nitrate and zinc sulfate solutions.
   - The student properly performs fecal flotations.

30) **The student uses correct methodology to perform fecal sedimentation to detect the presence of internal parasites.**
   - The student properly uses the sedimentation technique to detect ova or cysts that are too heavy to float in sodium nitrate solution, or those that could be distorted by sodium nitrate solution.
   - The student correctly performs a sedimentation method in which parasites will sink to bottom of a centrifuge tube.
   - The student shows awareness of the Baermann technique, for recovering nematode larvae (e.g., Strongyloides).

31) **The student uses correct methodology to perform direct smears to detect the presence of internal parasites.**
    - The student properly combines a small amount fresh fecal material with drop of normal saline solution on a slide and then places a cover slip over the mixture to create a very thin plane.
    - The student first scans the slide on 10× for large organisms, such as nematode larvae or Strongyloides. Next, the student observes the slide under 40× for bacteria, yeast, and/or protozoa, such as *Giardia* trophozoites and cysts.

32) **The student uses correct methodology to perform the centrifugation with flotation method for detecting the presence of internal parasites.**
    - As opposed to the simple flotation method, the student shows knowledge of the centrifugation with flotation method as the superior method for recovering parasite cysts (Hendrix and Robinson, 2012).
    - The student demonstrates understanding of the efficacy of this method for concentrating parasite ova, which float to the top and attach to the cover slip.
    - The student correctly performs the centrifugation with flotation method.

33) **The student accurately identifies parasitic nematodes commonly infecting domestic animals.**
    - The student shows knowledge of the life cycles of common nematodes.
    - The student demonstrates knowledge of the clinical significance of nematode infestations, including any potential zoonotic significance (e.g., cutaneous larva migrans, visceral larva migrans, and ocular larva migrans).
    - The student demonstrates knowledge of how to use the appropriate fecal flotation method to accurately identify nematode ova, such as those of Ascarids, *Ancylostoma* spp., *Uncinaria* spp., and *Trichuris* spp.
    - The student accurately identifies common adult nematodes as well as common nematode ova.

34) **The student accurately identifies trematodes commonly infecting domestic animals.**
    - The student shows knowledge of the life cycles of common trematodes.
    - The student demonstrates understanding of the clinical significance of trematode infestations, including any potential zoonotic significance.
    - The student demonstrates knowledge of how to use the appropriate method to detect common trematodes.
    - The student accurately identifies common trematodes, such as *Paragonimus* spp. and *Fasciola* spp.

35) **The student accurately identifies cestodes commonly infecting domestic animals.**
    - The student shows knowledge of the life cycles of common cestodes.
    - The student demonstrates understanding of the clinical significance of cestode infestations, including any potential zoonotic significance (e.g., *Echinococcus* spp.).
    - The student accurately identifies common cestodes, such as *Dipylidium* spp., *Taenia* spp., and *Echinococcus* spp.
    - The student displays knowledge of how to use the appropriate method to detect common cestodes.
    - The student accurately identifies adult cestodes and cestode ova.

36) **The student accurately identifies protozoa commonly infecting domestic animals.**
    - The student shows knowledge of the life cycles of common protozoa.
    - The student demonstrates knowledge of the clinical significance of protozoal infections, including any potential zoonotic significance (e.g., toxoplasmosis, etc.).
    - The student displays knowledge of how to use appropriate methods to detect common protozoa.
    - The student accurately identifies trophozoites and/or oocysts, such as those of *Giardia* spp., *Balantidium coli*, *Cryptosporidium* spp., and coccidia, including *Isospora* spp., *Eimeria* spp., and *Toxoplasma gondii*.

37) **The student correctly obtains representative specimens for microbiologic assessment.**
    - The student considers patient history and clinical findings in determining the collection procedure most appropriate to isolating the causative microorganism.
    - The student demonstrates awareness that, if at all possible, the specimen should be collected from the site of infection, since the sample must contain the causative organism to be of diagnostic value.
    - The student displays cognizance that samples should be collected prior to antimicrobial therapy, if at all possible.
    - The student takes all possible steps to minimize risks of sample contamination and maximize safety of personnel, including appropriate use of personal protective equipment (PPE).
    - The student uses aseptic technique when appropriate and collects a sufficient amount of the sample.
    - The student uses appropriate containers and keeps multiple samples separate from each other.
    - The student meticulously labels each sample and clearly indicates if a zoonotic microorganism is suspected.

38) **Using commercially prepared media and reagents, the student correctly cultures bacteria and performs sensitivity tests.**

- The student properly readies all equipment necessary for culturing bacteria and performing sensitivity tests. The student properly maintains all equipment, regularly checking temperatures of incubators and refrigerators.
- The student displays knowledge of appropriate uses of commercially available culture media, including, but not limited to enriched media, selective media, and differential media.
- The student correctly and aseptically inoculates culture media with bacteria. The student incubates cultures at optimal temperatures for appropriate time periods.
- The student follows proper protocols for antimicrobial susceptibility testing in accordance with the guidelines set forth by the Clinical and Laboratory Standards Institute (Veterinary Antimicrobial Susceptibility Testing (VAST) Subcommittee, 2015)
- The student correctly interprets antimicrobial susceptibility test results.

39) **Using commercially prepared media and reagents, the student participates in correctly identifying pathogens commonly affecting domestic animals.**

- The student shows knowledge of pathogens commonly infecting domestic animals, including their zoonotic potential.
- The student displays knowledge of various culture media and reagents and their appropriate uses.
- The student participates in following proper protocol when handling culture media and reagents.
- The student demonstrates the ability to identify bacteria based on growth characteristics, colony morphology, and other applicable factors.

40) **The student participates in the collection of milk samples and the performance of mastitis testing.**

- The student demonstrates knowledge of the significance of mastitis from an individual to a herd basis.
- The student displays knowledge of clinical signs of mastitis, while displaying awareness that mastitis may be subclinical.
- The student participates in the proper collection of milk samples, including cleaning the external surface of the teats appropriately and expressing a sample from each quarter.
- The student displays knowledge of the proper procedures for conducting mastitis testing and participates in it.
- The student correctly interprets the results of mastitis testing.

41) **The student demonstrates knowledge of and participates in correctly performing common biochemical tests for bacteria.**

- The student displays knowledge of appropriate uses of and participates in properly performing common biochemical tests for gram negative bacteria, including triple sugar iron (TSI) slants, urea slants, Simmon's citrate medium, motility agar, and so on.
- The student displays knowledge of appropriate uses of and participates in correctly performing diagnostic tests for gram positive bacteria, including bile-esculin media slants, mannitol salt agar (MSA), catalase test, and so on.
- The student correctly interprets the results of common biochemical tests for bacteria.

42) **The student demonstrates knowledge of and correctly performs staining procedures.**

- The student shows understanding of the differences in the biochemical composition of cell walls that result in differences in Gram staining reactions.
- The student correctly performs Gram staining procedures.
- The student accurately interprets results of Gram staining procedures, that is, differentiates Gram positive from Gram negative microorganisms. Based on Gram staining, the student displays the ability to identify morphology (e.g., cocci, bacilli, spiral) and arrangement (e.g., diplococci, staphylococci, or streptococci).
- The student displays understanding of the appropriate uses of acid-fast stains, particularly in revealing *Mycobacteria*. The student demonstrates awareness of the correct procedure to perform acid-fast stains, such as Kinyoun stain.

43) **The student demonstrates proper methodology for culturing dermatophytes and properly identifies the macroconidia of common dermatophytes.**

- The student shows familiarity with Sabouraud's dextrose agar as the standard medium for fungal cultures.
- The student demonstrates understanding of dermatophytosis as infection of keratinized tissue caused by *Microsporum*, *Trichophyton*, or *Epidermophyton* spp.
- The student displays knowledge of the clinical signs of dermatophytosis and its zoonotic potential.
- The student displays knowledge of dermatophyte test medium (DTM) as a selective and differential medium for dermatophytes that contains Sabouraud's dextrose agar, an antibacterial agent, cycloheximide (to inhibit saprophytic fungi), and a phenol red pH indicator.

- The student follows correct procedure for sample collection.
- The student correctly interprets the results of the DTM.
- The student shows cognizance that a color change after 10 days likely indicates a false positive due to contaminants.
- The student correctly performs microscopic cytology to identify common dermatophytes and differentiate them from contaminants. The student displays the ability to microscopically examine and accurately identify macroconidia.

44) **The student correctly obtains, prepares, and performs cytological evaluation of ear samples.**
- The student displays knowledge of ear canal anatomy of common domestic species.
- The student demonstrates knowledge of common pathogens of the external ear canal.
- The student shows knowledge of clinical signs of otitis.
- The student safely and properly obtains ear samples for cytology, culture, and antimicrobial susceptibility testing prior to cleaning and/or treatment, showing appreciation for the potential for ear pain associated with otitis.
- The student correctly prepares slides for microscopic evaluation.
- The student accurately evaluates ear cytology.

45) **The student participates in correctly obtaining, preparing, and assessing canine vaginal smears.**
- The student displays knowledge of the canine estrous cycle and common pathogens of the canine vagina.
- The student shows familiarity with indications for performing canine vaginal smears.
- The student participates in obtaining canine vaginal smears.
- The student accurately evaluates canine vaginal smears.
- The student participates in preparing the smear for microscopic evaluation.
- The student accurately evaluates canine vaginal smears.

46) **The student participates in performing prosection on a non-preserved animal, using all available precautions to minimize the risk of zoonotic disease.**
- The student demonstrates anatomical knowledge pertinent to postmortem examination.
- The student demonstrates awareness of the risk of infectious disease from tissue and/or fluids of deceased animals, regardless of whether or not patient was diagnosed with such disease.
- When handling necropsy specimens, the student shows the ability to apply knowledge of the transmission routes of zoonotic diseases.

- The student displays awareness of the extreme importance of personal protective equipment in performing a necropsy, including but not limited to a full-body apron, nitrile gloves, masks, and appropriate footwear.
- The student shows the ability to determine which tissue/fluid samples might be of greatest importance based on knowledge of the patient diagnosis at the time of death. At the same time, the student demonstrates understanding that samples from all major organs and other tissue, if diseased (e.g., oral cavity) and/or requested by veterinarian and/or pathologist should be harvested, as should relevant fluids (e.g., peritoneal, pleural, blood, ocular globe, etc.).
- The student displays knowledge of and participates in the proper procedure for performing a postmortem examination on a non-preserved animal.

47) **The student correctly obtains, stores, and ships specimens, following procedures required by the diagnostic laboratory.**
- The student shows awareness of the importance of collecting multiple samples from major organs and, when relevant, entire organs, such as kidneys or lymph nodes.
- The student displays knowledge that samples must be large enough to be sliced to allow slide preparation.
- The student displays knowledge that fluid samples should be retained either in capped, sterile syringes or in sterile vials as directed by the pathologist.
- The student displays knowledge that 10% neutral, buffered formalin is used for fixation of most tissue types and there should be a minimum of 10 parts of formalin to 1 part of tissue (Erhart, 1998).
- The student demonstrates awareness of potential risks of exposure to formalin that may occur while filling jars and placing samples, particularly its carcinogenic risks. The student displays knowledge of proper procedures for the safe handling of formalin containers.
- The student correctly places tissue samples in formalin jars of appropriate size, properly labeling them.
- The student displays knowledge of how to correctly gather all samples from the patient, either storing them for in-house use or packaging them according to requirements of the diagnostic laboratory. The student shows understanding that proper packaging is directed at preventing spillage or breakage and making certain the shipping box is appropriately labeled (e.g., indicating that contents are biological samples, indicating the top of the package and, when appropriate, any biohazard potential).

- The student wears nitrile gloves when handling specimens, even when they handling closed containers.
- The student demonstrates knowledge of how to and participates in properly packaging and shipping clinical specimens. The student shows awareness that individual courier companies should be contacted regarding specific packaging requirements, since these may differ from one courier to another.

48) **The student displays knowledge of how to safely handle rabies suspects and specimens.**
- The student demonstrates knowledge of the pathogenesis of rabies and the stages of the disease in the affected animal.
- The student displays knowledge of rabies transmission, as well as state and/or local regulations governing the handling of rabies suspects and specimens.
- The student shows awareness that any mammal that dies of unknown cause, as well as any animal that displayed signs of rabies in life, is treated as a rabies suspect.
- The student exhibits understanding that rabies is a zoonotic, reportable and fatal disease to animals and humans. Therefore, any person working with live or dead mammals should be immunized against rabies.
- The student displays understanding of state protocols that must be followed, including proper procedures for obtaining recommended human postexposure treatment, if there is any question regarding accidental exposure to tissues from a rabies suspect.
- The student displays knowledge of PPE that must be worn when obtaining samples from rabies suspects, including but not limited to face shields, waterproof gowns, full-length sleeves, and double gloves. The student shows knowledge that, after handling any samples from rabies suspects, all PPE must be shed and either disposed of in a biohazard container or submitted in a biohazard container to the laboratory for appropriate decontamination.
- The student shows knowledge that rabies can be definitively diagnosed only in isolated central nervous system tissue, particularly brain tissue. In small animal cases where the primary differential diagnosis is rabies, the entire head is removed from the body and shipped to the appropriate diagnostic laboratory. The student shows knowledge that the head should be shipped refrigerated (and never frozen); however, the appropriate state diagnostic laboratory should be contacted for specific instructions, since these may vary from state to state.
- The student displays knowledge that for large animal rabies suspects, some states require removal of the brain prior to submission to the diagnostic laboratory. Therefore, the appropriate state laboratory should be contacted for specific instructions (Van Winkle and Habecker, 2013).

References

American Heartworm Society. (2014a, July). *Current Canine Guidelines for the Prevention, Diagnosis and Management of Heartworm (*Dirofilaria immitis*) Infection in Dogs.* Retrieved February 26, 2016, from American Heartworm Society: www.heartwormsociety. org (accessed September 14, 2016).

American Heartworm Society. (2014b). *Summary of the Current Feline Guidelines for the Prevention, Diagnosis and Management of Heartworm (Dirofilaria immitis) Infection in Cats.* Retrieved February 26, 2016, from American Heartworm Society: www.heartwormsociety.org (accessed September 14, 2016).

Erhart, N. (1998). Proper biopsy procedure: collecting and handling tissue specimens. *Veterinary Technician*, 31–42.

Hendrix, C. M. and Robinson, E. (2012). *Diagnostic Parasitology for Veterinary Technicians* (4th edn). St. Louis: Elsevier.

Van Winkle, T. J., and Habecker, P. (2013). Basic necropsy procedures. In: J. M. Bassert, and J. A. Thomas, *McCurnin's Clinical Textbook for Veterinary Technicians* (8th edn). (pp. 561–582). Saunders.

Veterinary Antimicrobial Susceptibility Testing (VAST) Subcommittee. (2015). Retrieved February 26, 2016, from Clinical and Laboratory Standards Institute: csli. org (accessed September 14, 2016).

7

Radiography
Sandra Bertholf and Sabrina Timperman

1) **The student demonstrates and follows recommended procedures for radiation safety.**
   - The student acts in accordance with rules and regulations contained in Ionizing Radiation –Toxic and Hazardous Substances – Occupational Safety and Health Standards (United States Department of Labor, 1996).
   - The student shows awareness that the following individuals are not permitted in the radiography room during exposure: those less than 18 years of age, pregnant women, and unnecessary personnel.
   - The student shows awareness that manually restraining an animal for radiography should only be undertaken when all other forms of restraint are impossible or would be a significant health/safety risk to the patient. The student displays awareness that the best safety measure is refraining from being in the radiography room during exposure.
   - The student demonstrates knowledge of potential health dangers associated with radiation, maximum permissible doses (MPD) per year (whole body, individual tissues, and lens of eye), and the lifetime cumulative effects of radiation.
   - The student is familiar with the various types of personal protective equipment (PPE) and their proper applications and utilizes them appropriately.
   - The student wears appropriate PPE, including but not limited to lead apron, gloves, thyroid shield, badge, and lead safety glasses for every exposure. In addition, student displays awareness that all PPE must be worn correctly. For example, gloves must be worn properly; laying gloves on top of hands and arms is unacceptable.
   - The student demonstrates understanding of personal monitoring devices (dosimeter badges) and their purpose. The student appropriately wears and stores their dosimeter badge.
   - The student properly stores PPE. Gloves should be stored vertically on holders or lying flat with the ends propped open. Thyroid shields should be laid flat and lead safety glasses should be stored in a manner that prevents scratching or damage. Lead aprons should never be folded but instead draped over a rack.
   - The student displays awareness that PPE should be inspected routinely, radiographed at least yearly to detect defects, and the results properly documented. Defective PPE should be discarded and replaced.
   - The student wears their dosimeter badge correctly, positioning it outside the apron at the thyroid gland level. The student shows awareness that the dosimeter badge should be worn when in the facility. When not in use, the student makes certain to store the dosimeter badge in a place protected from exposure to radiation, heat, or chemicals.
   - The student displays knowledge of the limitations of PPE. In particular, the student demonstrates understanding that PPE helps provide protection from scatter radiation only, and does not protect against direct radiation. The student shows awareness that at no time should any part of their body be within the primary X-ray beam, even if wearing PPE.
   - The student demonstrates awareness of the importance of using proper collimation to reduce scatter radiation, thereby decreasing radiation exposure for personnel involved.
   - The student displays good judgement and takes all appropriate steps to minimize radiation exposure of personnel and patients.

2) **The student displays knowledge of how effective radiographic quality control procedures help to ensure production of diagnostic images.**
   - The student correctly defines the terms density and contrast and explains how they affect radiographic quality.

Assessing Essential Skills of Veterinary Technology Students, Third Edition. Edited by Laurie J. Buell, Lisa E. Schenkel and Sabrina Timperman.
© 2017 John Wiley & Sons, Inc. Published 2017 by John Wiley & Sons, Inc.
Companion website: www.wiley.com/go/buell/skills

- The student is able to evaluate whether or not radiographs are of diagnostic quality. The student determines if proper contrast and density have been achieved and demonstrates knowledge of how to adjust settings appropriately to acquire a quality image.
- The student displays awareness of how to record or appropriately log radiographic technique to help ensure continued quality images for that patient.
- The student displays knowledge of artifacts, their causes and how to correct them. For example, the student shows awareness that lack of contrast may be due to a light leak, radiation fog (exposure to undesired radiation), storage fog (heat and excess humidity), chemical fog (expired chemicals or excessive chemical temperature), expired film, improper technique, and so on.

3) **The student participates in developing and using a radiographic technique chart.**
   - The student displays awareness that every individual X-ray machine, whether conventional or digital, should have its own technique chart based on its unique features and that multiple technique charts may be necessary.
   - The student shows the ability to develop a technique chart, based on an understanding of milliamperage (mA), time (s), and kilovoltage peak (kVp). The student correctly uses Sante's rule to calculate kVp.
   - The student demonstrates the ability to use a technique chart to select correct settings for individual animals, depending on tissue thickness and the body part being radiographed.
   - The student carefully measures and positions patients, choosing appropriate radiographic techniques to minimize the need for repeat exposures.

4) **The student demonstrates the ability to properly position dogs, cats, and horses for radiographic studies.**
   - The student shows awareness of the correct views to obtain in order to properly visualize the area of interest.
   - The student demonstrates knowledge of pertinent canine and feline anatomy. The student correctly measures and positions dogs and cats for radiographic studies.
   - The student is able to define and properly demonstrate positioning terms such as lateral, ventrodorsal, dorsoventral, dorsopalmar, dorsoplantar, and craniocaudal.
   - The student correctly uses positioning aids and restraints, such as wedges, sandbags, tape, ties, cotton rolls, foam or plastic troughs, and so on, to position patients for diagnostic imaging.

- The student demonstrates proper patient handling and is aware of safety concerns associated with chemical and physical restraints, recognizing that the safety of both the patient and personnel are of the highest priority.
- The student displays knowledge of pertinent equine anatomy.
- The student demonstrates awareness of how beam distance and positional aspects affect equine radiography.
- The student shows knowledge of the potential for exposure to radiation when operating hand-held and/or portable radiographic equipment.
- The student demonstrates proper equine restraint techniques and is aware of safety precautions in handling injured horses, recognizing that the safety of both patient and personnel are of the highest priority.
- The student properly prepares an equine patient for a radiographic procedure. For example, when obtaining diagnostic images of the hoof, horseshoes should be removed and the lateral sulci of the frog packed with an appropriate material.
- The student demonstrates the ability to position the equine distal limb in a series of oblique, lateral, dorsopalmar, dorsoplantar and/or proximodistal ("skyline" view) positions.

5) **The student shows understanding of how to appropriately adjust radiographic techniques for exotic animal patients, including mice, rats, guinea pigs, lizards, and amphibians.**
   - The student displays understanding that, for most exotic species, measurements are often not used to calculate exposure factors; rather these are determined based on species and general size.
   - The student displays knowledge of normal exotic animal anatomy.
   - The student displays understanding that correct patient positioning is often achieved using anatomical landmarks rather than palpation.
   - The student shows awareness that positioning techniques for small rodents, lizards and amphibians differ depending on the type of radiographic equipment being used. For example, when using conventional or computed radiography (CR) systems, the patient is directly positioned on the radiographic cassette. The student displays knowledge of appropriate techniques for the type of X-ray machine being used and how to adjust kVp to reflect the small size of the patient.
   - The student displays understanding that while ideal positioning is often achieved by using sedation or anesthesia, patient status may preclude that option.

- The student displays understanding that using the fastest film-screen combinations and/or minimizing exposure time will aid in avoiding a blurry image due to movement.
- For lizards and amphibians, student demonstrates awareness that when using a conventional X-ray machine or a CR digital system, lateral radiographs should be taken using a horizontal beam at peak inspiration, since placing these species in lateral position distorts the lungs and diaphragm.

6) **The student properly operates stationary and portable X-ray units to radiograph live animals.**
   - The student properly utilizes radiographic equipment to create a diagnostic image.
   - The student displays knowledge of common radiographic procedures and chooses optimal positioning to obtain diagnostic radiographs.
   - The student demonstrates familiarity with different types of X-ray cassettes, their uses and care.
   - The student correctly selects an appropriate screen/cassette for a given procedure.
   - The student utilizes the Potter–Bucky Diaphragm properly.
   - The student demonstrates the ability to properly use portable units to obtain diagnostic radiographs.
   - The student follows procedures that maximize the safety of patient and personnel.

7) **The student produces quality diagnostic dental radiographic images**
   - The student properly positions the patient, film/sensor, and beam in the appropriate location to create a diagnostic image. For example, the student utilizes the parallel technique only for radiographing mandibular premolars and molars. The bisecting angle technique is utilized for radiographing all other teeth.
   - The student uses the correct film/sensor and placement.
   - The student properly adjusts the image by changing exposure time.
   - The student demonstrates the proper use of sandbags, bite blocks, V-shaped troughs, or any other type of positioning device needed to assist in increasing stability and correct placement.

8) **The student properly labels, files, and stores radiographic studies.**
   - The student stores images appropriately. For example, the student displays knowledge of the need to protect film from temperature extremes, ionizing radiation, and high humidity.
   - The student displays awareness that expired film should not be used because it will decrease image quality.

- The student properly handles both unexposed and exposed film, for example, handling film by the corners only.
- The student permanently labels images with required information including, but not limited to, patient identification, client identification, date, hospital and/or veterinarian's name, body part being radiographed, and positioning.
- The student files radiographic studies correctly and in an organized manner.

9) **The student properly completes radiographic logs, reports, files, and records.**
   - The student properly logs, and files radiographic studies, completing all necessary documentation.
   - The student correctly records information of the radiographic study in the patient's medical record.

10) **The student participates in utilizing either positive or negative contrast agents in performing a GI series, pneumocystogram, excretory urogram (intravenous pyelogram), or other radiographic contrast study.**
    - The student displays knowledge of various contrast agents, their uses, and correct routes and sites of administration.
    - The student correctly calculates doses of contrast agents.
    - The student shows awareness of potential common adverse effects associated with various contrast studies and contrast agents. For example, dehydration should be corrected before performing an excretory urogram to decrease the risk of potential renal damage.
    - The student closely monitors patients during and following a contrast study.
    - The student shows knowledge of how to accurately time and properly label images when performing a GI series or excretory urogram.
    - The student shows knowledge of how to properly use air as a contrast medium when performing a negative contrast study such as a pneumocystogram.

11) **The student participates in correctly performing radiographic screening for canine hip dysplasia (CHD).**
    - The student demonstrates knowledge of the multifactorial pathophysiology of canine hip dysplasia, including its genetic roots, the influence of nutritional factors and its prevalence in certain breeds.
    - The student explains the importance of only breeding dogs with acceptable certification but is aware that this does not guarantee that offspring will not have CHD.

- The student is aware of the minimum age requirement for accurate CHD evaluation in relation to the specific technique being used.
- The student shows familiarity with Orthopedic Foundation for Animals (OFA) and PennHIP techniques, their relative advantages and disadvantages and the different requirements for each.
- The student displays knowledge of how to properly position a dog for radiographic evaluation for CHD, explaining why proper positioning is crucial and how improper positioning can lead to a non-diagnostic image.
- The student is aware that general anesthesia is required for accurate PennHIP evaluation and deep sedation or anesthesia is recommended for accurate OFA evaluation.
- The student differentiates between diagnostic and non-diagnostic images. The student shows familiarity with rating scales for OFA and PennHIP techniques.

12) **The student displays knowledge of correct care and maintenance of radiographic equipment and is able to recognize when it is defective.**
- The student demonstrates knowledge of basic principles regarding how radiographic equipment operates.
- The student demonstrates awareness of the need for routine scheduled maintenance to ensure consistent quality diagnostic imaging.
- The student demonstrates knowledge of how to properly identify defective radiographic equipment. For example, when the collimator light is nonfunctional, proper field size cannot be assessed.
- The student recognizes when it is necessary for the manufacturer to service the equipment.
- The student demonstrates familiarity with common artifacts, their causes, and how to correct and prevent them.

Reference

United States Department of Labor. (1996, June 20). Retrieved from Occupational Safety and Health Administration: www.osha.gov/pls/oshaweb/owadisp.show_document?p_table=STANDARDS&p_id=10098 (accessed September 14, 2016).

8

Laboratory Animal Care and Procedures
Natalie H. Ragland

1) **The student displays understanding of the need for the use of laboratory animals in biomedical research.**
   - The student shows appreciation of the importance of upholding ethical, humane, and scientific standards in the use of laboratory animals.
2) **The student displays working knowledge of federal, state, local, and institutional animal welfare regulations as they apply to laboratory animal research.**
   - The student demonstrates working knowledge of the content of the *Guide for the Care and Use of Laboratory Animals* (National Research Council, 2011).
   - The student demonstrates understanding of the importance of the IACUC (Institutional Animal Care and Use Committee) as it pertains to laboratory animal medicine and research (National Research Council, 2011; Fox, Anderson, Leow, and Quimby, 2002).
   - The student displays understanding of the IACUC member's responsibilities and functions in research settings, which include (National Research Council, 2011; Fox, Anderson, Leow, and Quimby, 2002; Suckow and Schroeder, 2010).
     - Assessing facility operations and procedures
     - Reviewing research protocols
     - Ensuring institutional compliance
     - Reviewing methods to improve animal health and welfare
     - Supporting the 3 Rs (Replacement, Reduction, Refinement).
3) **The student correctly identifies and properly restrains rodents (mice, rats) and rabbits.**
   - The student correctly identifies and differentiates mice, rats, and rabbits.
   - The student correctly restrains adult and weanling mice by using one hand to grasp the base of the tail while the other hand is scruffing the neck. (American Association of Laboratory Animal Science (AALAS), 2014a,b; Danneman, Suckow, and Brayton, 2013).

   - The student correctly restrains mice using rubber tipped forceps by grasping the loose skin around the neck region or close to the base of the tail (AALAS, 2014a,b; Danneman, Suckow, and Brayton, 2013).
   - The student correctly restrains rats by using one hand to grab the base of the tail closest to the rump while placing the other hand over the back of the rat and simultaneously using the thumb and forefinger to press the forelegs near the head (AALAS, 2014a,b; Sharp and Villano 2013).
   - The student properly restrains rabbits, making certain to support their hindquarters. The student demonstrates knowledge of the rabbit's susceptibility to injury if improperly restrained, particularly its tendency to kick and sustain bone fractures. The student displays understanding that rabbits are never to be handled by the ears. (AALAS 2014a,b; Suckow and Schroeder, 2010).
   - The student recognizes the various restraint devices used in laboratory animal medicine for rodents (mice, rats) and rabbits. (AALAS, 2014a,b; Suckow, and Brayton, 2013; Sharp and Villano, 2013; Suckow and Schroeder, 2010).
4) **The student correctly determines the sex and demonstrates knowledge of the reproduction of rodents (mice, rats) and rabbits.**
   - The student correctly identifies rodent gender via comparing the anogenital distance (distance between the genital papilla and anus) and the lack of grossly visible nipples in males (AALAS, 2014a,b; Danneman, Suckow, and Brayton, 2013; Sharp and Villano, 2013).
   - The student displays awareness that the doe (female rabbit) often has a narrow head and a large dewlap (skin fold that hangs around the neck) at the caudal *mandibulocervical* region (under the chin) and that the buck (male rabbit) lacks a dewlap and generally have larger heads (AALAS, 2014a,b; Suckow and Schroeder, 2010).

Assessing Essential Skills of Veterinary Technology Students, Third Edition. Edited by Laurie J. Buell, Lisa E. Schenkel and Sabrina Timperman.
© 2017 John Wiley & Sons, Inc. Published 2017 by John Wiley & Sons, Inc.
Companion website: www.wiley.com/go/buell/skills

- Based on accurate knowledge of anatomy, the student demonstrates the proper technique to sex a rabbit by using gentle pressure with the thumb and forefinger around the genital area to allow visibility of genitalia, while observing for the opening of the organ (AALAS, 2014a,b; Suckow and Schroeder, 2010).
- The student displays knowledge of estrous cycles, breeding characteristics, gestation periods, parturition, and litter sizes of mice, rats, and rabbits (Fox, Anderson, Leow, and Quimby, 2002; AALAS, 2014a,b; Danneman, Suckow, and Brayton, 2013; Sharp and Villano, 2013; Suckow and Schroeder, 2010). For example, based on accurate knowledge of physiology, the student displays understanding:
  - That female mice and rats are in estrus every 4–5 days, whereas rabbits are induced ovulators.
  - That the presence of a copulatory (vaginal) plug is an indication of mating in mice and rats.
  - That the gestation period for mice is 12–19 days, for rats it is 21–23 days and for rabbits it is 31–32 days.
  - Of the definition of the Whitten effect.
  - That the buck is always taken to the doe's cage for mating
  - That does pull fur from their chests and abdomens to create nest boxes in preparation for kits (newborn rabbits).

5) **The student demonstrates proper handling of rodents and rabbits**.
- The student correctly grasps and handles mouse pups by picking up a group of pups together, gently grasping the skin near and around their shoulder blades or by cupping hands around the body (AALAS, 2014a,b; Danneman, Suckow, and Brayton, 2013).
- The student correctly handles adult/weanling mice using rubber tipped forceps or fingertips by grasping the loose skin around the neck region or close to the base of the tail (AALAS, 2014a,b; Danneman, Suckow, and Brayton, 2013).
- The student correctly handles adults/weanling rats by using one hand to grab the base of the tail closest to the rump while placing the other hand over the back of the rat and simultaneously using the thumb and forefinger to press the forelegs near the head. (AALAS, 2014a,b; Sharp and Villano, 2013).
- The student correctly transports rats by placing a hand around the thorax and abdomen, taking care not to squeeze the thorax.
- The student safely and effectively picks up rabbits by using one hand to scruff the nape of the neck and the other hand to support the hindquarters (AALAS, 2014a,b; Suckow and Schroeder, 2010).

When carrying a rabbit long distances, the student makes certain that the rabbit's head is nestled in the bend of the elbow and the hindquarters are supported.

6) **The student shows knowledge of proper diets for laboratory rodents and rabbits based on their unique nutritional requirements**.
- The student shows knowledge that for adult laboratory rabbits, commercial nutritionally balanced rabbit pellets comprise the mainstay of the diet, supplemented with grass hays (e.g., Timothy hay), alfalfa cubes, and fresh greens, such as lettuces, parsley, carrots, broccoli, cabbage, and so on (AALAS, 2014a,b; Suckow and Schroeder, 2010)
- The student shows knowledge that a proper diet for adult rats and mice consists of commercial nutritionally balanced rat/rodent pellets *which may vary in fat and protein content depending on study protocols* (AALAS, 2014a,b; Fox, Anderson, Leow, and Quimby, 2002).

7) **The student provides appropriate, species-specific food, water, and enrichment**.
- The student checks daily to ensure that *ad lib* fresh water is provided in clean sipper tubes or bottles.
- For rats and mice, the student provides appropriate rodent pellets *ad lib* unless otherwise specified by the research IACUC protocol.
- For laboratory rabbits, the student provides appropriate rabbit pellets (*ad lib) and provides scheduled supplemental feed unless otherwise specified by the research IACUC protocol.*
- The student displays knowledge of the purpose of enrichment given to mice and rats and provides appropriate enrichment, such as Nestlets, Nylabones®, Mouse Igloos®, Enviro-dri®, and housing huts.
- The student displays knowledge of the purpose of enrichment given to rabbits and provides appropriate enrichment, such as ropes, balls, Nylabones®, and nest boxes.

8) **The student displays knowledge of how to perform identification procedures in mice, rats, and rabbits.**
- The student displays understanding of identification systems for mice, rats and rabbits as well as which systems are appropriate for use in each species (AALAS, 2014a,b; Danneman, Suckow, and Brayton, 2013; Sharp and Villano, 2013; Suckow and Schroeder, 2010).
- The student shows knowledge of how to perform identification procedures, including ear notching/punching/tagging, tattooing, and microchipping and applying permanent dye (AALAS, 2014a,b; Danneman, Suckow, and Brayton, 2013; Sharp and Villano, 2013).

- The student displays awareness that toe clipping should only be performed on neonatal mice. (AALAS, 2014a,b; Danneman, Suckow, and Brayton, 2013).

9) **The student properly performs subcutaneous injections in mice, rats, and rabbits.**
   - The student demonstrates knowledge of the maximum volume that can be administered subcutaneously (Fox, Anderson, Leow, and Quimby, 2002; AALAS, 2014a,b; Danneman, Suckow, and Brayton, 2013; Sharp and Villano, 2013; Suckow and Schroeder, 2010).
   - With the animal properly restrained, the student correctly places the needle into the loose skin of the scruff (between the skin and underlying muscle in the hypodermis) and slowly injects the solution (AALAS, 2014a,b; Danneman, Suckow, and Brayton, 2013; Sharp and Villano, 2013; Suckow and Schroeder, 2010).

10) **The student participates in properly performing an intraperitoneal injection in the mouse.**
    - The student demonstrates knowledge of the maximum volume that can be administered intraperitoneally to mice (AALAS, 2014a,b; Danneman, Suckow, and Brayton, 2013).
    - The student correctly describes how to administer drugs intraperitoneally in the mouse, injecting lateral to midline into the caudal right quadrant of the abdomen (AALAS, 2014a,b; Danneman, Suckow, and Brayton, 2013).
    - The student participates in correctly restraining the mouse for intraperitoneal injection and/or performing the injection.

11) **The student participates in correctly collecting IV blood samples from the rat.**
    - The student correctly describes how to obtain blood from the tail vein of the rat, using the "warm tail technique" to promote vasodilation (AALAS, 2014a,b; Suckow and Schroeder, 2010; Sharp and Villano, 2013).
    - The student participates in properly restraining the rat for IV blood collection and/or performing venipuncture.

12) **The student correctly collects IV blood samples from the rabbit.**
    - The student properly obtains blood samples from rabbits using the lateral/marginal ear vein, the lateral saphenous vein and/or the central ear artery (AALAS, 2014a,b; Suckow and Schroeder, 2010).
    - The student displays awareness that sedation may be required for individual rabbits, particularly if large amounts of blood must be collected (AALAS, 2014a,b; Suckow and Schroeder, 2010).

13) **The student participates in properly performing oral dosing in rats and mice.**
    - The student demonstrates knowledge of pertinent anatomy in rodents, including structures of the oral cavity, esophagus, and stomach (Fox, Anderson, Leow, and Quimby, 2002; AALAS, 2014a,b; Danneman, Suckow, and Brayton, 2013; Sharp and Villano, 2013; (Suckow and Schroeder, 2010).
    - The student shows awareness of potential dangers of administering medications to species that cannot vomit (Fox, Anderson, Leow, and Quimby, 2002; AALAS, 2014a,b) (Danneman, Suckow, and Brayton, 2013; Sharp and Villano, 2013; Suckow and Schroeder, 2010).
    - The student displays appreciation of the importance of measuring a sufficient distance from the mouth to the sternum (AALAS, 2014a,b).
    - The student participates in properly inserting a gavage tube and administering drugs to rodents by this route (AALAS, 2014a,b).
    - The student demonstrates familiarity with dosing syringes, feeding tubes, and metal balling guns (AALAS, 2014a,b; Danneman, Suckow, and Brayton, 2013; Sharp and Villano, 2013; Suckow and Schroeder, 2010).

14) **The student displays functional knowledge of anesthetic and recovery procedures in rats, mice, and rabbits.**
    - In general, the student demonstrates basic knowledge of appropriate uses, major contraindications, common adverse effects, and appropriate routes and methods of administration for injectable and inhalant anesthetic, preanesthetic and/or analgesic agents commonly used in rats, mice, and rabbits, including the use of tribromoethanol (Avertin®) in rodents (Fox, Anderson, Leow, and Quimby, 2002; Danneman, Suckow, and Brayton, 2013; Sharp and Villano, 2013).
    - The student demonstrates knowledge of how to administer an injectable agent to induce anesthesia in mice, rats and rabbits and how to maintain anesthesia by administering an inhalant anesthetic via face mask or nose cone (AALAS, 2014a,b; Danneman, Suckow, and Brayton, 2013; Sharp and Villano, 2013; Suckow and Schroeder, 2010).
    - The student shows awareness that, in general, food, and water should not be withheld prior to surgery in rats, mice, and rabbits. Since rodents and rabbits are coprophagic, however, some recommend a shortened period of removal of feed before certain procedures to allow for sufficient gastric emptying (Danneman, Suckow, and Brayton, 2013; Sharp and Villano, 2013; Suckow and Schroeder, 2010).

- The student displays awareness of the need to apply ophthalmic lubricant in rodents and rabbits (Danneman, Suckow, and Brayton, 2013; Sharp and Villano, 2013; Suckow and Schroeder, 2010).
- The student displays knowledge of how to monitor anesthesia in rats, mice and rabbits, properly checking respiratory and cardiovascular parameters, body temperature, muscle tone, and reflexes (e.g., palpebral, pedal, pinna, corneal, etc.) (Fox, Anderson, Leow, and Quimby, 2002; Danneman, Suckow, and Brayton, 2013; Sharp and Villano, 2013; Suckow and Schroeder, 2010).
- The student displays knowledge of how to recognize and address anesthetic overdose, hypothermia, hypotension, and other common anesthetic complications (Fox, Anderson, Leow, and Quimby, 2002; Danneman, Suckow, and Brayton, 2013; Sharp and Villano, 2013; Suckow and Schroeder, 2010).
- The student demonstrates knowledge of appropriate thermoregulation devices (Fox, Anderson, Leow, and Quimby, 2002).
- The student demonstrates knowledge of appropriate postoperative care, including common analgesics given to rodents and rabbits following surgical procedures (Fox, Anderson, Leow, and Quimby, 2002; Fox, Anderson, Leow, and Quimby, 2002; Danneman, Suckow, and Brayton, 2013; Sharp and Villano, 2013; Suckow and Schroeder, 2010).
- The student displays knowledge of up-to-date guidelines for avoiding, minimizing and alleviating pain in laboratory animals. The student displays understanding of how to recognize pain and/or distress in rats, mice, and rabbits and demonstrates knowledge of how to implement appropriate pain management protocols, while continuing to monitor the animal's ongoing status. The student demonstrates awareness that any animal given anesthetic and/or analgesic agents must be closely monitored for adverse effects in the pre-anesthetic, anesthetic, and post-procedural periods (Fox, Anderson, Leow, and Quimby, 2002; AALAS, 2014a,b; Danneman, Suckow, and Brayton, 2013; Sharp and Villano, 2013; Suckow and Schroeder, 2010).

15) **The student accurately identifies and describes common signs of the following diseases in laboratory mice and demonstrates knowledge of which diseases are zoonotic.**
(Fox, Anderson, Leow, and Quimby, 2002; AALAS, 2014a,b; Danneman, Suckow, and Brayton, 2013).

a) **Viral**
- Adenovirus types 1 and 2 (MAV1 and 2)
- Mouse minute virus (MVM)
- Epizootic diarrhea of infant mice (EDIM)

b) **Bacterial**:
- *Cilia-Associated Respiratory Bacillus* (CAR)
- *Klebsiella* spp.
- *Pasturella* spp.
- *Staphylococcus* spp.
- *Pseudomonas aeruginosa*
- *Proteus* spp.

c) **Parasitic**
- *Syphacia obvelata* (Pinworm)
- Giardia
- *Myobia musculi* and *Mycoptes musculinus* (mite infestation).

16) **The student accurately identifies and describes common signs of following diseases in laboratory rats and demonstrates knowledge of which diseases are zoonotic.**
(Fox, Anderson, Leow, and Quimby, 2002; AALAS, 2014a,b; Sharp and Villano, 2013).

a) **Viral**:
- Adenovirus
- Mouse minute virus (MVM)
- Rotavirus

b) **Bacterial**
- *Corynebacterium*
- *Streptococcus* spp.
- *Pseudomonas aeruginosa*
- *Staphylococcus* spp.
- *Proteus* spp.

c) **Parasitic**
- *Syphacia muris* (Pinworm)
- *Radforia ensifera* (mite infestation)
- Entamoeba

17) **The student accurately identifies and describes common signs of following diseases in laboratory rabbits and demonstrates knowledge of which diseases are zoonotic.**
(Fox, Anderson, Leow, and Quimby, 2002; AALAS, 2014a,b; Suckow and Schroeder, 2010).

a) **Viral**
- Rotavirus

b) **Bacterial**
- *Pasturella multocida*
- *Clostridium piliforme* (Tyzzer disease)
- *Clostridium difficile*

c) **Parasitic**
- Oxyuriasis (Pinworm)

d) **Mycotic**
- *Trichophyton mentagrophyte* (Ringworm).

e) **Other**
- Gastric trichobezoar.

References

American Association of Laboratory Animal Science (AALAS). (2014a). *Assistant Laboratory Animal Technician Training Manual.* Memphis: McNeal Graphics.

American Association of Laboratory Animal Science (AALAS). (2014b). *Laboratory Animal Technician Training Manual.* Memphis: McNeal Graphics.

Danneman, P., Suckow, M., and Brayton, C. (2013). *The Laboratory Mouse* (2nd edn). Boca Raton: CRC Press.

Fox, J. G., Anderson, L. C., Leow, F. M., and Quimby, F. W. (2002). *Laboratory Animal Medicine* (2nd edn). San Diego: Academic Press.

National Research Council. (2011). *Guide for the Care and Use of Laboratory Animals* (8th edn). Washington, DC: National Academy Press.

Sharp, P., and Villano, J. (2013). *The Laboratory Rat* (2nd edn). Boca Raton: CRC Press.

Suckow, M., and Schroeder, V. (2010). *The Laboratory Rabbit* (2nd edn). Boca Raton: CRC Press.

9

Avian and Exotic Animal Nursing

Sabrina Timperman, Lisa E. Schenkel, Laurie J. Buell and Carol J. Gamez

1) **The student properly demonstrates understanding of and performs safe and effective restraint methods for birds.**
   - The student displays knowledge of pertinent avian anatomy and physiology.
   - To help ensure the safety of the patient and handler, the student demonstrates understanding of the need for specialized restraint techniques for birds.
   - The student displays appreciation of the importance of minimizing stress in birds and shows knowledge of signs of stress in birds, such as fluffing of feathers, open-beak breathing, and tail bobbing.
   - The student displays the ability to properly restrain birds, grasping around the head, and never grabbing the body or squeezing the chest (pectoral area). For small birds, the student gently holds the head between the thumb and the forefinger or the middle finger and supports the lower limbs. The student shows awareness that a second handler may be needed to restrain the wings and body of larger birds.

2) **The student demonstrates understanding of and displays the ability to provide client education on particular diets/nutritional concerns for birds, reptiles, amphibians, guinea pigs, hamsters, gerbils, and ferrets.**
   - The student displays knowledge of how the physiology of each species determines its nutritional needs.
   - The student displays knowledge that the proper diet for birds depends on species. The student also shows awareness that feeding an all seed diet is not recommended for captive birds as it causes a deficiency in vitamin A (Greenacre and Gerhardt, 2010).
   - The student demonstrates awareness that based on order and species, reptiles require widely varying diets, ranging from carnivorous to omnivorous to herbivorous.
   - The student demonstrates awareness that insectivorous reptiles and amphibians eating crickets or mealworms require "gut-loading" diets year round (a diet of crickets alone is nutritionally inadequate and unacceptable). To determine proper diets for each class, order, and species, the student displays knowledge of appropriate references to consult, such as *Fowler's Zoo and Wild Animal Medicine* (Fowler and Miller, 2014).
   - Regarding guinea pigs, the student demonstrates knowledge that the recommended diet for pet guinea pigs consists of guinea pig pellets and free choice high quality grass hay. The student also shows awareness that leafy greens contain high levels of Vitamin C as well as calcium and should be offered in small amounts.
   - The student displays awareness that guinea pigs need daily vitamin C supplementation (approximate daily requirements for adults are 10–25 mg/kg daily for maintenance and 30 mg/kg during pregnancy) (Hawkins and Bishop, 2012).
   - The student displays awareness that the vitamin C contained in commercial pellets expires 90 days after date of manufacture. The student also shows awareness that in order to assure adequate vitamin C activity, drinking water that is supplemented with vitamin C must be changed daily (vitamin C is quickly degraded by light and substances that may be found in water) (Hawkins and Bishop, 2012).
   - Regarding hamsters, the student demonstrates knowledge that nutritionally balanced pelleted feed or rodent blocks with at least 16% protein and 4–5% fat are recommended with small amounts of fruits and vegetables making up no more than 10% of the total diet) (Harkness, Vandewoude, Turner, and Wheler, 2010). The student demonstrates awareness that hamsters in the wild are omnivorous.
   - Regarding gerbils, the student displays awareness that commercial gerbil pellets with at least 16–22%

Assessing Essential Skills of Veterinary Technology Students, Third Edition. Edited by Laurie J. Buell, Lisa E. Schenkel and Sabrina Timperman.
© 2017 John Wiley & Sons, Inc. Published 2017 by John Wiley & Sons, Inc.
Companion website: www.wiley.com/go/buell/skills

protein, along with some leafy greens, are recommended, but seed mixes are not nutritionally adequate and not recommended (Harkness, Vandewoude, Turner, and Wheler, 2010).

- Regarding ferrets, the student demonstrates awareness that, since they are strict carnivores, a whole prey diet is the ideal. However, because this is not an acceptable option for many ferret owners, the student displays knowledge that ferrets may be fed commercial dry kibble diets, containing at least 30–35% protein and approximately 15–20% fat. The ingredients label should list high quality meat products as the first three ingredients (Hawkins and Bishop, 2012).
- The student shows knowledge of the consequences of feeding each species an inappropriate and/or inadequate diet.
- The student explains the nutritional needs and the proper diets for birds, reptiles, amphibians, guinea pigs, hamsters, gerbils, and ferrets clearly and succinctly and in a manner understandable to the client.
- The student recommends appropriate references such as texts, educational websites, and clinical education materials.

3) **The student demonstrates understanding of and displays the ability to provide client education regarding the particular water needs of birds, reptiles, amphibians, guinea pigs, hamsters, gerbils, and ferrets.**
   - The student displays knowledge of how the physiology of each species determines its water needs and how each species obtains water in its natural environment.
   - The student demonstrates awareness, depending on the species, that adequate fresh water, cleaned daily or more frequently, should be available at all times.
   - The student displays knowledge that some birds, in addition to drinking water, require a bird bath that should be emptied, cleaned, and refreshed daily.
   - The student demonstrates awareness that amphibians and some reptiles also require bathing/basking pools that should be emptied, cleaned, and refreshed daily.
   - The student displays knowledge that, for guinea pigs, hamsters, gerbils, and ferrets, adequate amounts of fresh water should be available in sipper bottles that are checked for proper function and cleaned daily. The student demonstrates awareness that the sippers of such bottles may become clogged even though they appear to be functioning.
   - The student explains water needs for birds, reptiles, amphibians, guinea pigs, hamsters, gerbils, and ferrets clearly and succinctly, and in a manner understandable to the client.

- The student recommends appropriate references such as texts, educational websites, and clinical education materials.

4) **The student demonstrates understanding of and displays the ability to provide client education regarding the particular caging/aquarium needs of birds, reptiles, amphibians, guinea pigs, hamsters, gerbils, and ferrets.**
   - The student shows familiarity with the importance of: (1) exposing the bird to fresh air and unfiltered sunlight (and/or a full spectrum UV light source) at least 20 minutes twice weekly; (2) misting the bird frequently to encourage grooming and hydration; and (3) providing the opportunity for a water bath or shower.
   - The student shows understanding that birds require cages that are as large as possible; at minimum, the cage should be large enough to allow the bird to spread its wings without touching the sides. The student demonstrates awareness that the cage should be frequently cleaned (to remove organic debris) and disinfected with a dilute solution of chlorine bleach and water only. The student displays awareness that many other household cleansers should not be used because they may emit fumes that are toxic to birds, and that even when a dilute solution of chlorine bleach and water is used, the bird should be out of the cage until the fumes have evaporated.
   - The student displays familiarity with appropriate cage substrates and perches of varying diameter (i.e., to help prevent chronic inflammatory conditions of the foot or bumblefoot), and the need to replace substrates and perches frequently (i.e., when soiled).
   - The student demonstrates awareness that, since natural habitats of reptiles and amphibians vary widely, housing should mirror the natural environment as closely as possible (including light, temperature, humidity, ventilation, etc.). The student displays knowledge of appropriate references to consult for the proper environment, caging/aquarium, and caging substrate for each class, order, and species.
   - The student demonstrates awareness of the importance of exposing reptiles to full spectrum UV light for the appropriate time period depending on species.
   - The student shows knowledge that exposure to direct sunlight is ideal (i.e., exposure to sunlight through glass is inadequate). The student also displays awareness that the UVB output of full spectrum UV lamps needs to be measured periodically in order to determine if the lamp no longer emits

adequate UVB light and needs to be replaced (Stephen and Fleming, 2014).

- The student displays knowledge that some amphibians are highly susceptible to water toxins and pH changes (due to skin permeability), necessitating daily skin inspections. The student also shows awareness that some lungless amphibians depend on cutaneous respiration (Wilson, 2010).
- For ferrets, guinea pigs, hamsters, and gerbils, the student displays knowledge of appropriate caging, cage substrates, lighting, ventilation, cage size, and the need to provide accessories and/or materials for nesting, climbing, exercising, and/or hiding.
- The student demonstrates awareness that cages or pens for ferrets must be large enough for exercise and should include a "den" area in which to hide. In addition, when outside of their cages or pens, ferrets should not be left unsupervised and, due to their propensity to chew almost anything, the home should be "ferret-proofed" (Pye, 2003). The student displays awareness that ferrets may be trained to use litter boxes.
- The student displays knowledge that aquaria or metal cages with solid floors are suitable for guinea pigs because of their very soft feet, which are prone to injury. The student shows knowledge that appropriate cage substrates include newspaper, shredded paper, or clean straw (Quesenberry, Donnelly, and Mans, 2012). In addition, the student displays awareness that for hamsters and gerbils, hardwood chips, or recycled paper pellets are suitable cage substrates, but synthetic, commercial nesting materials are not recommended because they may injure the feet or cause impaction if ingested.
- The student displays awareness that guinea pigs enjoy being housed with other guinea pigs, but hamsters and gerbils are best housed singly.
- The student explains caging/aquarium needs for birds, reptiles, amphibians, guinea pigs, hamsters, gerbils, and ferrets clearly and succinctly in a manner understandable to the client.
- The student recommends appropriate references such as texts, educational websites, and clinical education materials.

5) **The student demonstrates understanding of and displays the ability to provide client education regarding reproduction of birds, reptiles, amphibians, guinea pigs, hamsters, gerbils, and ferrets.**
   - In general, the student demonstrates familiarity with species-specific breeding requirements, including environmental and dietary adjustments necessitated by pregnancy and/or lactation.
   - The student displays knowledge of the anatomy and physiology of reproduction in the various species.

- The student demonstrates awareness of how to sex various species and their specific breeding requirements.
- The student displays knowledge of common causes and clinical signs of dystocia in the various species, such as improper nutrition. For example, a cockatiel on an all seed diet is at high risk for becoming egg bound due to hypocalcemia.
- The student shows appreciation for the complications of dystocia and the need for immediate veterinary attention.
- The student displays knowledge that some birds have difficulty laying eggs and many of these are first time egg layers. In addition, the student shows awareness that certain species are more prone to becoming chronic egg layers leading to an increased risk for hypocalcemia and egg binding.
- The student displays knowledge that the presence of a male is not necessary to stimulate egg laying behavior in a female bird.
- The student shows awareness that the presence of a male is not necessary for egg production in some species of reptiles and amphibians.
- The student demonstrates awareness that reptiles can be egg-laying or viviparous. The student shows familiarity with the proper temperature and humidity for egg incubation and clinical signs of "egg-bound" females.
- The student displays awareness that amphibians can be oviparous, viviparous, and ovoviviparous (Klaphake, 2010).
- The student demonstrates knowledge that guinea pigs breed best in monogamous pairs, but pregnant sows must be separated from other adults until the litter is weaned. The student shows awareness that guinea pigs are prone to dystocia due to narrow pelvic canals, pups that tend to be larger in size, and fusion of the pelvic symphysis. Sows bred after 8–12 months have a higher incidence of dystocia (Hawkins and Bishop, 2012).
- The student shows knowledge that hamsters should be bred by placing the female in the male's cage one hour before dark and removing her after mating or when fighting ensues. The student displays awareness that cannibalism of the young is common in hamsters; however, fostering and hand-raising of the young is not recommended.
- The student shows awareness that gerbils are non-seasonally polyestrous and prefer monogamous pairing, with the male helping to raise the young (Harkness, Vandewoude, Turner, and Wheler, 2010).
- The student displays knowledge that intact female ferrets, or jills, are induced ovulators with a 39–42-day gestation period (Powers and Brown, 2012).

The student shows understanding that females that are not intended to be bred should be spayed because if not bred, females usually remain in heat, which can cause a fatal, estrogen-induced anemia (Powers and Brown, 2012).

- The student explains pertinent reproduction for birds, reptiles, amphibians, guinea pigs, hamsters, gerbils and ferrets clearly and succinctly in a manner understandable to the client.
- The student recommends appropriate references such as texts, educational websites, and clinical education materials.

6) **The student demonstrates understanding of and displays the ability to provide client education on the particular grooming needs of birds, reptiles, amphibians, guinea pigs, hamsters, gerbils, and ferrets.**

- The student demonstrates knowledge of proper techniques for beak, wing and nail clipping. The student shows awareness of the goal of wing clipping as prevention of sustained flight as opposed to making the bird unable to fly (Tully Jr., 2014).
- The student demonstrates knowledge that reptiles vary greatly in grooming requirements. For example, the student displays awareness that in reptiles other than snakes and most chelonians, nail trimming on a regular basis is advisable. In addition, the student demonstrates understanding that handling of reptiles should be avoided during shedding (ecdytic), and excessively low humidity is associated with dysecdysis (Cheek, Richards, and Crane, 2010).
- The student shows awareness that clouding of eyes in reptiles is an indication of impending shedding.
- The student demonstrates knowledge that small mammals have varying needs for basic grooming. For example, ferrets may require ear-cleaning, toenail trimming and dental prophylaxis. As another example, because the incisors and molars of guinea pigs grow continuously, the teeth may require trimming.
- The student shows awareness that guinea pigs may need toenail trimming, and long-haired breeds need brushing.
- The student explains basic grooming for birds, reptiles, amphibians, guinea pigs, hamsters, gerbils, and ferrets clearly and succinctly in a manner understandable to the client.
- The student recommends appropriate references such as texts, educational websites, and clinical education materials.

7) **The student demonstrates understanding of and displays the ability to provide client education regarding the proper transportation methods for birds, reptiles, amphibians, guinea pigs, hamsters, gerbils, and ferrets.**

- The student displays ability to describe appropriate transportation methods for various species, based on the knowledge that stress of inappropriate travel methods can seriously affect patient health.
- The student displays knowledge of appropriate methods for transporting birds, with awareness that they should be protected from excessive heat or cold and not left unattended in cars.
- The student demonstrates awareness that reptiles and amphibians should be transported either in their own caging/aquaria or in a similar, but more compact, enclosure that contains some substrate and is kept covered and warm, protected from temperature extremes and not left unattended in a car. In addition, the student displays knowledge that amphibians should be lightly misted with warm water prior to transport.
- The student shows knowledge that rodents may be transported in their own cages (or smaller cages, if their usual habitats are too large), and a sheet or towel may be used to cover the cage in order to reduce visual stressors. The student demonstrates knowledge that the cage should be protected from excessive heat or cold and not left in an unattended car.
- The student demonstrates awareness that ferrets may be transported safely in cat carriers.
- The student explains appropriate transportation methods for birds, reptiles, amphibians, guinea pigs, hamsters, gerbils, and ferrets clearly and succinctly in a manner understandable to the client.
- The student recommends appropriate references such as texts, educational websites, and clinical education materials.

8) **The student demonstrates knowledge of and displays the ability to provide client education regarding the clinical role of proper husbandry in maintaining the well-being of the birds, reptiles, amphibians, guinea pigs, hamsters, gerbils, and ferrets.**

- The student shows awareness that the majority of disease states in these species are due to improper husbandry.
- The student recognizes inappropriate husbandry of the various species such as improper nutrition and environment.
- The student displays knowledge of normal behavior patterns of the various species. The student displays ability to recognize abnormal behavior patterns.
- The student explains the clinical role of proper husbandry for birds, reptiles, amphibians, guinea pigs,

hamsters, gerbils, and ferrets clearly and succinctly in a manner understandable to the client.

- The student recommends appropriate references such as texts, educational websites, and clinical education materials.

9) The student collects objective data in birds in the form of an avian exam.

- Prior to beginning the physical exam, the student observes the bird's behavior and appearance in the cage. In addition, the student accurately determines the respiratory rate and character while the bird is at rest.
- The student chooses the appropriate method for weighing the bird based on the bird's behavior and condition and obtains an accurate weight.
- The student uses appropriate restraint techniques.
- The student correctly examines the head, displaying awareness that the top of the head should be smooth (matted feathers may be a sign of illness), eyes should be clear and open, and touching the medial canthus should cause a blink reflex. The student checks the eyes for symmetry, discharge or redness and gently lifts the eyelid to subjectively monitor for hydration as the lid resumes its normal location.
- The student properly examines the cere and nostrils, displaying knowledge that the cere should be smooth and soft, the nostrils should be clear, free of discharge and symmetrical, and the operculum within the nares should be free of abnormal accumulation. The student correctly locates and examines the ears by gently parting the feathers on each side of the head. The student shows awareness that the beak should be smooth, shiny, and of normal length. The student then properly inserts an oral speculum to examine the oral cavity, assessing the choanal slit and its papillae, as well as the color and moistness of the oral mucosa. The student palpates the crop for abnormalities.

- The student observes and accurately determines the respiratory rate during restraint, showing understanding that, after examination, a healthy bird should resume its pre-handling respiratory rate within minutes. The student displays awareness that respiratory rates and heart rates are faster in smaller birds than larger birds. Using a pediatric stethoscope, the student auscultates the heart, accurately determining the heart rate.
- The student displays understanding of and the ability to correctly determine the "body condition score." The student properly palpates the pectoral muscles and abdomen.
- The student properly examines the cloaca and everts it, if possible, to examine the cloacal mucosa. The student correctly examines the uropygial gland in birds that have one.
- The student properly examines the feathers over the entire body, as well as the skin of the feet, also checking the nails for overgrowth.

10) The student correctly performs an avian nail trim.

- The student displays knowledge of the nail anatomy of common avian species.
- The student correctly restrains the bird for the nail trim.
- The student demonstrates the ability to properly hold both guillotine and scissors-type nail clippers, Dremel Motor Tools or files; estimates the location of vascular matrix; correctly trims nails and applies cauterization agents/hemostatic techniques, when needed.

References

Cheek, R., Richards, S., and Crane, M. (2010). Snakes. In: B. Ballard, and R. Cheek, *Exotic Animal Medicine for the Veterinary Technician* (pp. 119–165). Ames: Wiley-Blackwell.

Fowler, M. E., and Miller, R. E. (2014). *Zoo and Wild Animal Medicine Current Therapy*. Philadelphia: W.B. Saunders Company.

Greenacre, C. B., and Gerhardt, L. (2010). Psittacines and passerines. In: B. Ballard, and R. Cheek, *Exotic Animal Medicine for the Veterinary Technician* (pp. 11–43). Ames: Wiley-Blackwell.

Harkness, J. E., Vandewoude, S., Turner, P. V., and Wheler, C. L. (2010). *Harkness and Wagners Biology and Medicine of Rabbits and Rodents*. Ames: Wiley-Blackwell.

Hawkins, M. G., and Bishop, C. R. (2012). Disease problems of guinea pigs. In: K. E. Quesenberry, and J. W. Carpenter, *Ferrits, Rabbits, and Rodents Clinical Medicine and Surgery* 3rd edn). (pp. 295–310). St. Louis: Elsevier.

Klaphake, E. (2010). Reproductive disease in reptiles and amphibians. *American Board of Veterinary Practition Symposium 2010 Proceedings Online*. Denver: American Board of Veterinary Practitioners.

Lennox, A. M., and Bauck, L. (2012). Small rodents: Basic anatomy, physiology, husbandry, and clinical techniques. In: K. E. Quesenberry, and J. W. Carpenter, *Ferrits, Rabbits, and Rodents Clinical Medicine and Surgery* (3rd edn) (pp. 339–353). St. Louis: Elsevier.

Powers, L. V., and Brown, S. A. (2012). Ferrets: Basic anatomy, physiology and husbandry. In: K. E. Quesenberry, and J. W. Carpenter, *Ferrets, Rabbits, and Rodents Clinical Medicine and Surgery* (pp. 1–12). St. Louis: Elsevier.

Pye, G. (2003). Ferrit basics. *Proceedings of the North American Veterinary Conference, Vol. 17* (pp. 1257–1258). Gainesville: Eastern States Veterinary Association.

Quesenberry, K. E., Donnelly, T. M., and Mans, C. (2012). Biology, husbandry and clinical techniques of guinea pigs and chinchillas. In: K. E. Quesenberry, and J. W. Carpenter, *Ferrets, Rabbits, and Rodents Clinical Medicine and Surgery* (pp. 279–294). St. Louis: Elsevier.

Stephen, B. L., and Fleming, G. J. (2014). Current herpetologic husbandry and products. In: D. R. Mader, and S. J. Divers, *Current Therapy in Reptile Medicine and Surgery* (pp. 2–12). St. Louis: Elsevier.

Tully Jr., T. N. (2014). Care of birds, reptiles, and small mammals. In: J. M. Bassert, and J. A. Thomas, *McCurnin's: Clinical Textbook for Veterinary Technicians* (8th edn) (pp. 810–843). St. Louis: Elsevier.

Wilson, B. (2010). Amphibians. In B. Ballard, and R. Cheek, *Exotic Animal Medicine for the Veterinary Technician* (2nd edn) (pp. 205–237). Ames: Wiley-Blackwell.

Index

a

Abscesses. *See* Wounds and abscesses
Activated clotting time (ACT)   52
Admitting and discharging
      patients   1
Ambu® bag. *See* Resuscitation bag
American Society of
      Anesthesiologists (ASA)
      classification of patient
      physical status   25
Amphibians
   egg laying in   71
   nutrition of   69
   radiographic techniques   61
   transportation of   72
Anal sac expression, canine   13
Anesthesia and analgesia   25–30
   analgesic therapy. *See* Pain
      management
   anesthetic monitoring. *See*
      Anesthetic, monitoring
   endotracheal intubation. *See*
      Endotracheal intubation
   in laboratory animals   65–66
   pain assessment. *See* Pain
   preanesthetic period   49–51
   perioperative management 25–30.
      See also Anesthetic risk,
      evaluation of
Anesthetic and analgesic agents   2,
      6, 7, 20, 26–27, 29, 32, 38, 65,
      66. *See also* Anesthetic,
      complications and
      emergencies
   administration of   5–7, 30, 42
   adverse effects   29, 42
   dosage calculations   39, 42
   efficacy of   28, 29
Anesthetic equipment   30–34
   anesthetic machines and breathing
      circuits   32, 33

oxygen, administration of
      20, 21
   positive pressure ventilations,
      administration of   21, 29, 33
   monitoring equipment   20, 27–28,
      30, 40
   operation and maintenance
      of   27, 28
Anesthetic
   complications and
      emergencies   29–30
   induction   26–27, 45
   logs   14, 54
   monitoring   22, 25, 30. *See also*
      Anesthetic, complications and
      emergencies
   records   42
   regimens (protocols)   40
   risk, evaluation of   25, 26
Animal Medicinal Drug Use
      Clarification Act
      (AMDUCA)   7
Aquarium needs   70–71
Aseptic technique,
   in administering injectable
      medications   7, 15
   in intravenous catherization   18
   in operating room   46
   during surgery   40, 41
   in urethral catheterization   12
Auscultation of heart and lungs   18,
      27, 28, 73
   cat   11
   cow   11
   dog   11
   horse   11
Autoclave, operation and
      maintenance   45
Avian
   caging   70–72
   client education   69–73

egg laying   71
grooming needs   72
importance of proper husbandry
      72–73
nail trimming   73
nursing   69–73
nutrition   69
physical examination   73
restraint   10, 69
transportation   72
water needs   70

b

Babesiosis   53
Bacteria
   biochemical tests for   55
   culturing   55–56
   identification of pathogenic   55
   staining procedures for   55
Baermann technique   53
Balling gun, use of   16
Bandage(s)
   during postoperative period   43
   and splints   19, 21
Basic life support (BLS)   20
Bathing and applying dips
      12–13
Biologics
   laws and regulations governing   7
   safety concerns when working
      with   7
Bird. *See* Avian
Blood chemistry testing   52
Blood coagulation   52
Blood collection. *See also*
      Venipuncture
   from laboratory rabbits and
      rats   65
Blood films
   evaluation of   51
   preparation and staining of   51

Assessing Essential Skills of Veterinary Technology Students, Third Edition. Edited by Laurie J. Buell, Lisa E. Schenkel and Sabrina Timperman.
© 2017 John Wiley & Sons, Inc. Published 2017 by John Wiley & Sons, Inc.
Companion website: www.wiley.com/go/buell/skills

Blood parasites. *See Dirofilaria* spp.;
    Haemobartonella spp
Blood pressure monitors   28, 33–34
Blood transfusion   19
Bovine.*see* Cattle
Bradycardia   30
Breeding and reproduction
    procedures   13
    see also Reproduction
Breeds, recognition of   9
Buccal mucosal bleeding time   52

c

Cages   9, 70–71
    encaging and removal from   9
    labeling   9
Canine hip dysplasia (CHD)   61
Capnography   21, 31
Capnometry   31
Cardiopulmonary arrest (CPA)   20
Cardiopulmonary resuscitation
    (CPR)   19–21
Castration, surgical   37
Catheterization, intravenous   15,
    17–18, 20
    cephalic   17–18
    jugular   11
    saphenous   11–12
Catheterization, urinary
    care and maintenance   12
    of female dog   12
    of male cat   12
    of male dog   12
Cats
    catheterization of   12
    cystocentesis   12
    ear cleaning   13
    hand-pilling   16
    intramuscular injections   15
    intravenous injections   15
    nail trimming   13
    onychectomy in   38
    orchiectomy   37–39
    otic medications   13
    ovariohysterectomy in   37, 39
    radiographic positioning   60
    restraint of   9
    subcutaneous injections   15
    voided urine sampling   12
Cattle
    dehorning   38
    halter   10
    shute   10
    tail restraint   10

Cautery   41
Central venous pressure (CVP)   18
Cephalic vein
    IV catheterization   17–18
    venipuncture   11
Cesarean section   37
Cestodes, parasitic, identification
    of   54
Client education   3, 17, 22, 69–73
Clinical laboratory
    instruments and equipment   49
    management   49–50
    quality control methods   49
    safety   49
Clinical status, monitoring of   27–28
Cold sterilization   42, 45
Communication skills   1, 3. *See also*
    Client education
Complete blood count (CBC)   50
Computer skills   2, 41
Conduct
    professional   1, 49
    operating room. *See* Operating
        room conduct
Confidentiality   4
Consent forms   1, 39
Controlled drugs. *See* Scheduled
    (controlled) drugs
Crash cart, emergency   19, 30
Crisis intervention   3
Crossmatch testing   19
Culturing of bacteria   55
Cystocentesis   12
Cytological evaluation
    of canine vaginal smears   56
    collection of samples for   11, 12
    of ear samples   56

d

Dehorning in cattle and goats   38
Dental
    at-home care   22–23
    procedures in small
        animals   21–23
    prophylaxis   22
    radiography   22, 61
    tooth identification   21–22
Dermatophyte test medium
    (DTM)   55–56
Dermatophytes
    culturing   55
    identification of   55–56
Diagnostic sample
    collection

    for ear cytology   11
    of fecal samples   11
    for vaginal cytology   11
    preparation and handling
        12, 59
Diet(s) *see* Nutrition; Nutritional
    requirements
Dirofilaria spp., identification of
    52, 53
    heartworm antigen kit test   53
Discharge instructions   43–44
Dogs
    anal sacs, expressing   13
    canine hip dysplasia (CHD)   61
    cystocentesis   12
    ear cleaning   13
    hand-pilling   16
    intramuscular injections   15
    intravenous injections   15
    muzzles   9
    nail trimming   13
    onychectomy in   38
    orchiectomy in   37–39
    otic medications   13
    ovariohysterectomy in   37, 39
    prolapse of nictitans gland
        in   38
    radiographic positioning   60
    restraint of   9
    subcutaneous injections   15
    urine sampling   12
    vaginal smears   56
    voided urine sampling   12
Doppler devices   34
Dosage calculations. *See* Drug(s),
    dosage calculations
Dose syringe, use of   16
Dosimeter badges   59
Drug administration   5–7, 15–16,
    19–21, 26, 28
    appropriate routes and methods
        for   5, 6
    emergency   26, 30
    enteral   6, 15
    hand pilling dogs and cats   16
    by injection. *See* Injection
    in laboratory animals   65
    ophthalmic medications   16–17
    oral, in laboratory animals   65
    preparation of drugs for   7
    topical   16
    use of balling gun   16
    use of dose syringe   16
    use of stomach (gastric) tube   16

Drug(s) 5–8
  administration, fundamentals 5–7
  adverse reactions to 5–8, 13, 19, 26, 29, 30, 32, 42, 65
  anesthetic and analgesic. *See* Anesthetic and analgesic agents
  categories 5
  dispensing 8
  disposal of 2, 6
  dosage calculations 5–7, 25, 26, 39, 42–43
  emergency 19, 26, 30
  labels 7–8
  laws and regulations governing 2, 7
  mechanisms of action 5
  medication orders 5, 7
  over-the-counter (OTC) 7
  preparation 7
  prescription 7
  reconstitution 5, 16
  safety concerns when working with 7, 8
  scheduled substances 2, 6–7, 26, 30
  therapeutic uses and responses 5, 6
Dystocia 38, 71

e
Ears
  cleaning and applying medication to 13
  cytology 11
  samples 56
E-collars 10, 43, 44
Egg laying
  in amphibians 71
  in birds 71
  in reptiles 71
Ehrlichiosis 53
Electrocardiography (ECG) 21, 31–32
ELISA 52
Elizabethan collars 10, 43, 44
Encaging small animals 9
Endotracheal intubation 27
  anesthesia 32
  dental procedures 22
Enema administration 17
Enrichment, laboratory 64
Enteral administration. *See* Drug administration, enteral

Equine *see* horses
Esophageal stethoscope 31
Ethics and jurisprudence 3–4. *See also* Laws and regulatory agencies
Euthanasia 3
Excretory urogram (intravenous pyelogram) 61
Exotic animals
  caging/aquarium 70–72
  grooming needs 72
  importance of proper husbandry 72–73nursing 69–73
  nutrition 69–72
  radiographic techniques 60–61
  reproduction 71–72
  transportation 72
  water needs 70

f
Face masks 32, 44
Fasting 26
Fecal
  centrifugation with flotation method 54
  direct smear 56
  flotation 53, 54
  sampling 11
  sedimentation 53
Feline *see* Cats
Ferrets
  grooming needs 72
  nutrition 70
  reproduction in 71–72
  transportation of 72
Fiber optic equipment 41–42
Fibrinogen assay 52
Filing
  radiographic images 61
  systems 2
Financial transactions 2
First aid 19
Fleas 53
Flies 53
Fluid therapy
  administration of 17, 18
  calculations 18
  delivery systems 18–19
  monitoring hydration status 18
  perioperative period 43
  subcutaneous administration of 17
Food additives 14

Food and Drug Administration (FDA), role of 7, 14
Forms, preparation of 1
  from dog 11
  from horse 11
  from rabbit 65
  from rat 65

g
Gastric intubation 16
Gerbils
  grooming needs of 72
  housing 70, 71, 73
  importance of proper husbandry 72–73
  nutrition 69–72
  reproduction 71–72
  transportation 72
  water needs 70
GI series 61
Gloves, surgical 42, 44
Goats, dehorning of 38
grooming
  in birds and exotic animals 72
  in small animals 12–13
Guinea pigs
  dystocia in 71
  grooming needs in 72
  housing 70, 71
  nutrition 69, 70
  reproduction in 71, 72
  transportation 72

h
Haemobartonella spp., identification of 52
Halters and leads, affixing to horses and cattle 10
Hamsters
  caging 70–72
  nutrition in 69
  reproduction in 71
  transportation 72
  water needs 70
Hand-pilling 16
Hazardous materials disposal of 2, 7
Hazards, laboratory 49
Heart sounds. *See* Auscultation of heart and lungs
Heartworm. *See Dirofilaria* spp
Hematocrit 50
Hematologic indices. *See* Red blood cell indices

Hemoglobin determination   50
Hip dysplasia, canine   61
Horses
  anesthesia   28
  dose syringing   16
  intramuscular injections   15
  intravenous injections   15
  radiographic positioning   60
  restraint and leading   10
  tail and leg wraps   13
  twitching   10
Husbandry
  avian   72–73
  of common domestic
      species   12–14
  of exotic animals   72–73
  see also under individual animal
Hygiene, laboratory   49
Hypotension during anesthesia   30
Hypothermia during peri-anesthetic
      period   30
Hypoventilation   31

i
Identification techniques
  of laboratory animals   9, 64–65
  permanent   13
  surgery and   39
Injections   15
  intramuscular   15
  intraperitoneal (in laboratory rats
      and mice)   65
  intravenous   6, 15
  subcutaneous   15, 65
Interpersonal (interactive) skills   3
Intravenous blood samples
  from cat   11
  from cow   11
  from rabbits   65
  from rodents   65
Intravenous pyelogram   61
Ionizing Radiation –Toxic and
      Hazardous
      Substances – Occupational
      Safety and Health
      Standards   59
Isolation units   2
Ixodes spp., 53

j
Jugular vein, venipuncture   11

k
Keratoconjunctivitis sicca (KCS)   16

l
Labeling
  of diagnostic samples   12
  drug   7, 8
  laboratory samples   49
  patient identification   9
  radiographic images   61
Laboratory animals   63–66
  anesthesia and analgesia in. *See*
      Anesthesia and analgesia
  blood collection from   65
  common conditions and diseases
      in   66
  drug administration to   65
  feeding and watering   64
  handling and restraint   64
  identification techniques in   9,
      64–65
  nutritional needs of   64
  pain management   66
  reproduction of   63–64
  use of, in biomedical research   63
  welfare regulations   63
Laboratory, clinical. *See* Clinical
      laboratory
Laparotomy   38
Laryngoscope   34
Laws and regulatory agencies   2, 3,
      6–8, 30, 57, 59, 63
  Drug Enforcement Agency
      (DEA)   6–7
  Food and Drug Administration
      (FDA)   2, 7, 14
  US Department of Agriculture
      (USDA)   2, 7
Lice   52
Lizards, radiographic techniques
      in 61
Logs   2, 26, 49
  anesthetic/surgical   14, 54
  laboratory   2
  of radiographic studies   2, 60
  scheduled (controlled)
      substances   6
Lung sounds. *See* Auscultation of
      heart and lungs

m
Management. *See* Veterinary
      management
Masks   32
  surgical   44
Mastitis testing   55
Medical nursing   9–23

Medical record keeping   1, 2
  anesthetic   42
  pulse   10–11
  radiographic   61
  respiratory rate   11
  surgical   39, 42
  temperature   10
Medication(s). *See* Drug(s)
Mice
  intraperitoneal injection in   65
  oral dosing in   65
Microbiology
  bacterial pathogens. *See* Bacteria
  culture media and reagents   55
  dermatophytes. *See* Dermatophytes
  sample collection in   54
  sensitivity (antimicrobial
      susceptibility) tests   55
Microchips   9
Microfilaria detection   53
Microorganism collection   54
Milk sampling   55
Mites   52
Modified Knotts test   53
Muzzles   9

n
Nail trimming
  of birds   73
  of cats   13
  of dogs   13
  of small mammals   72
  of reptiles   72
Necropsy
  performing post-mortem
      examinations   56
  rabies suspects and specimens, safe
      handling of   57
  sample collection, storing and
      shipping   56
Nematodes, parasitic, identification
      of   54
Neonatal (newborn) care
  nursing of   14
  temperature of   25
Nociception assessment   28
Nursing, medical. *See* Medical nursing
Nursing, surgical. *See* Surgical
      nursing
Nutrition
  hospital protocols   14–15
  postoperative, rodents and
      rabbit   66
  therapeutic   14

Nutritional requirements
    amphibians 69
    birds 69
    of common domestic species 14–15
    ferrets 70
    gerbils 69–70
    guinea pigs 69
    hamsters 69
    of laboratory rodents and
        rabbits 64
    in postoperative period 43
    reptiles 69
    species-specific 64
Nutritional supplements 14

o
Ocular diagnostic tests 16–17
    fluorescein staining 16–17
    Schirmer tear test 16
    tonometry 16–17
On-line veterinary services 2
Onychectomy 38
Operating room. *See also* Aseptic
        technique
    cleaning and maintenance
        of 46–47
    conduct 41
Oral cavity, evaluation of 21, 73
Oral dosing. *See* Drug administration,
        enteral
Orchiectomy 37–39
Organs, exposed, care of 41
Orthopedic Foundation for Animals
        (OFA) 62
Orthopedic procedures 37
Otitis 56
Ovariohysterectomy 37, 39
Oxygen sources 33

p
Packaging
    of diagnostic samples 12
    of laboratory samples 49
Packed cell volume (PCV) 50
Pain behavior 28–29
Pain
    assessment of 27–29, 42
    management (analgesic
        therapy) 29, 42–43, 66
        See also Anesthetic and analgesic
            agents
    perception 28–29
    physiological effects of 29
    scales 29

Parasites, internal, detection 53–54
Partial thromboplastin time
        (PTT) 52
Patient evaluation
        (assessment) 9–12
    of common domestic
        species 9–12
    peri-anesthetic assessment 39–40
Patient history 10
Patient identification. *See*
        Identification
PennHIP 62
Personal protective equipment
        (PPE) 2
    in laboratory 49
    microorganisms and 54
    in performing necropsy 56
    in rabies 57
    in radiography 59
Pesticides
    disposal of 2, 7
    laws and regulations governing 7
    safety concerns when working
        with 7
Pharmacotherapeutics 15–21
Pharmacy 9–13
    orders 11
Physical examination, avian 73
Platelet (thrombocyte) count 51
Pneumocystogram 61
Poisonous plants, common 14
Positioning, patient
    radiographic 60–62
    during surgery 40
Prolapsed organ, correction of 38
Prothrombin time (PT) 52
Protozoa, parasitic, identification
        of 54
Pulse oximetry 28, 30–31, 33
Pulse taking 10–11

q
Quality control
    laboratory equipment 49
    radiography 59–60

r
Rabbits
    intravenous blood samples 65
    laboratory enrichment 64
    handling 64
    nutrition 64
    restraint of 63
    sex determination of 63–64

Rabies suspects and specimens 57
Radiographic equipment. *See also*
        X-ray film
    automatic processor, operation
        of 61
    care and maintenance of 62
    X-ray units, operation of 61
Radiographic screening for canine
        hip dysplasia. *See* Hip
        dysplasia, canine
Radiography 59–62
    canine hip dysplasia screening 62
    contrast media in 61
    dental 22, 61
    logs/reports/files/records 61
    positioning and restraint
        for 60–62
    quality control in 59–60
    safety 59
    stationary and portable X-ray
        units 61
    storage of radiographic
        studies 61
    technique adjustment for exotic
        animal patients 60–61
    technique chart development
        in 60
Rats
    intravenous blood samples 65
    oral dosing in 65
RECOVER CPR initative (2012) 20,
        21
Rectal temperature taking 34
Recumbent patient, care of 19
Red blood cell count 50–51
Red blood cell indices 51
Refractometry 50
Reproduction
    avian 71
    in common domestic species 13
    ferret 71–72
    gerbil 71
    guinea pig 71, 72
    hamster 71
    in laboratory rabbits, rats and
        mice 63
    rabbit 63
    reptile and amphibian 71
Reptiles
    egg laying in 71
    grooming needs of 72
    nutrition in 69
    shedding in 72
    transportation of 72

Restraint
  of birds 10, 69
  of cats 9, 13, 16
  of cows 10, 16
  of dogs 9, 10, 13
  of horses 10, 13, 16, 60
  of laboratory rodents and
     rabbits 63
  pole 10
Resuscitation (Ambu®)) bag 21,
    30, 33
Reticulocyte count 51
Risk
  anesthetic 25, 26
  radiation dosages 59
Rocky Mountain Spotted Fever 53
Rodents
  laboratory enrichment 64
  handling of 64
  nutrition in 64
  restraint of 63
  sex determination of 63–64
  transportation of 72
  see also under types
Route of administration
  anesthetics 26–27
  drug 6
Ruminants
  dose syringing 16
  intravenous injections 15
  subcutaneous injections 15

S
Safety
  assessment of veterinary
     patient 9
  laboratory 49
  substances 7
Sanitation procedures 2, 13
Saphenous veins
  IV catheterization 17–18
  venipuncture 11–12
Sarcoptes 52
Scavenging systems. *See* Waste gas
    scavenging systems
Scheduled substances 2, 6–7,
    26, 30
Scheduling appointments and
    procedures 1
Serologic assays 52
Sex determination of laboratory
    rodents and rabbits 63–64
Sharps, disposal of 49

Skin scrapings 17
Slide/card agglutination
    tests 52
Snap tests 52
Staining
  of blood films 51
  fluorescein 16–17
  procedures 55
Sterilization, methods of 45
  cold 42, 45
  gas 45
Storage
  cytology 12
  of laboratory samples 49,
    56–57
  radiographic images 61
Subcutaneous injections 15, 65
Suction devices, during surgery 41
Surgical
  assisting 37–47
  care of exposed tissue in 41
  clean-up, post-procedural. *See*
    Operating room, cleaning and
    maintenance
  equipment, and facilities
    management 44–47. *See also*
    Autoclave
  instrument
    nomenclature and uses 44
    passing 41
    packs 44
    preparation of 44
  gowns, masks, gloves and drapes,
    preparation of 42, 44
  nursing 37–47
  patient evaluation and
    preparation 39–44
  patient positioning 42
  procedures 39
  records 39, 42
  skin preparation 40
Suture
  materials and needles 45–46
  removal 44

t
Tail docking 38
Tattoos 9
Temperature 10
  during peri-anesthesia 30
  monitoring devices, during
    anesthesia 34
  neonates 25

Thrombocyte estimation 51
Ticks 53
Tissues, exposed, care of 41
Topical medications 16
Total protein concentration in
    plasma 50
Toxins and poisons 14
Tracheostomy 21
Transportation
  of birds 72
  of diagnostic samples 12
  of laboratory samples 56–57
  of reptiles and amphibians 72
  of rodents 72
  transportation 72
Trematodes, parasitic, identification
    of 54

u
Urinalysis 39
Urinary bladder palpation 40
Urine sample collection
  cystocentesis in dog and cat 12
  urinary catheterization. *See*
    Catheterization, urinary
  voided urine of dog and cat 12
Urine testing 49–50
Uterine prolapse 38

v
Vaccination certificates 1, 2
Vaccines and vaccination 5
Vaginal cytology 11
Vaginal smears, canine 56
Venipuncture
  of canine cephalic vein 11
  of canine jugular vein 11
  of canine saphenous vein
    11–12
  of equine jugular vein 11
  of feline cephalic vein 11
  of feline jugular vein 11–12
  of ruminant jugular vein 11
Ventilation(s)
  monitoring adequacy of 28, 29,
    31, 33
  positive-pressure 21, 29, 30, 33
Veterinary management 1–4
  admitting and discharging
    patients 1
  bookkeeping procedures 2
  communication skills 1, 3
  computer skills 1–2, 41

ethics   3–4
filing   2, 61
grief management skills   3
inventory control   2, 6, 7
professional demeanor and
   conduct   1, 3, 49
sanitation procedures. *See*
   Sanitation procedures
scheduling appointments and
   procedures   1
triaging emergency patients   1
veterinarian–client–patient
   relationship   3
Veterinary teamwork   3

Veterinary terminology   1, 7
Vocalization, pain and   28

W
Waste gas scavenging systems   33
Watering
   birds   70
   guinea-pigs   69
   laboratory animals   64
   reptiles and amphibians   70, 72
   small mammals   70
Welfare regulations of laboratory
   animals   63
White blood cell count   50, 51

Wound(s)
   and abscess care   19, 21, 40, 43–44
   postoperative care of   43

X
X-ray film
   labeling, filing and storing   61
   processing of   61

Z
Zoonotic diseases
   in laboratory mice   66
   in laboratory rats   66
   in laboratory rabbits   66